Juliette and the Mystery Bug

JULIETTE

AND THE MYSTERY BUG

By Colleen & Terry Shepherd

Illustrated by Casey Ratchford

For
Juliette
and
Hudson

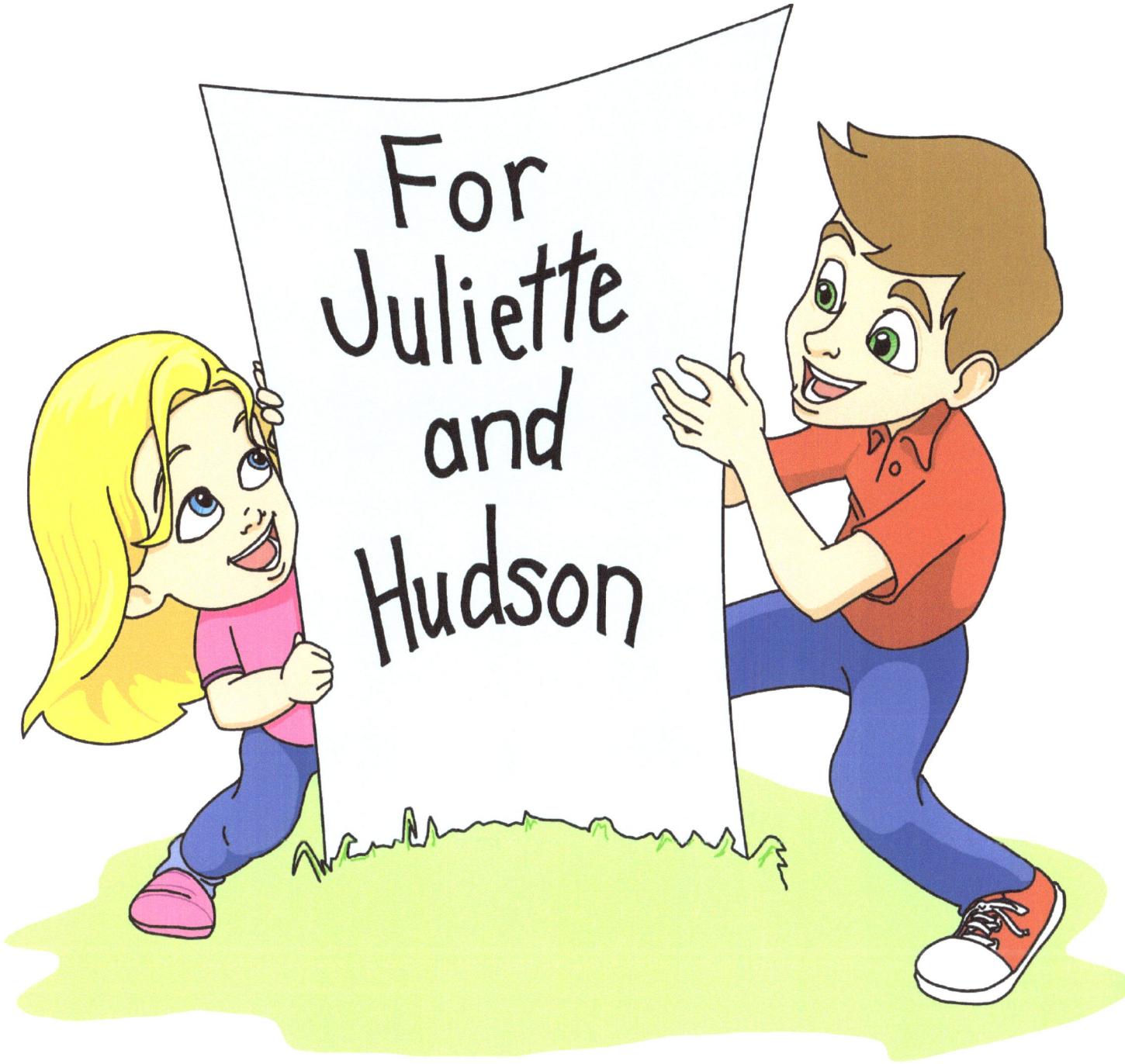

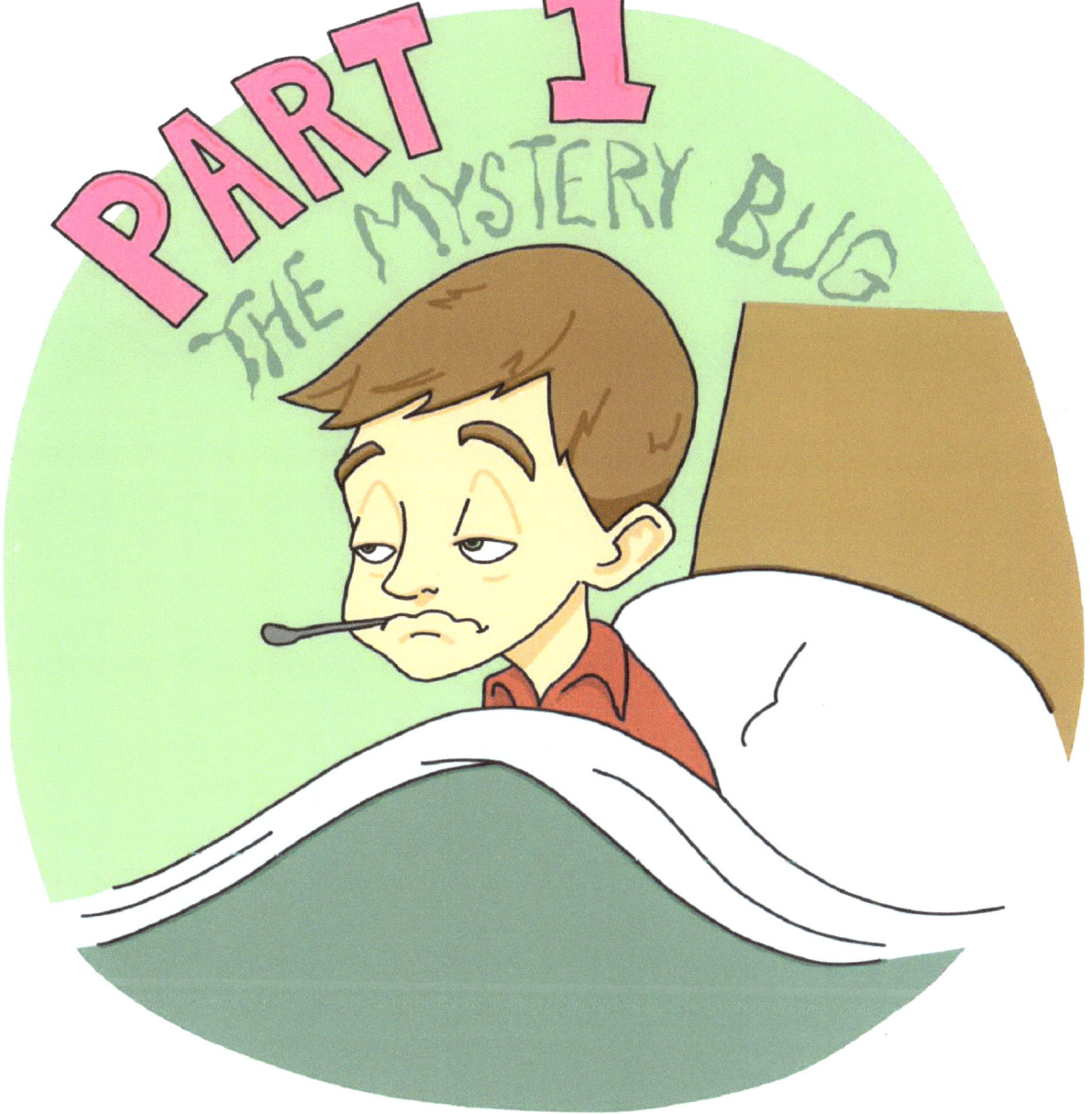
PART 1
THE MYSTERY BUG

It began on a Monday.
She heard Hudson sneeze.

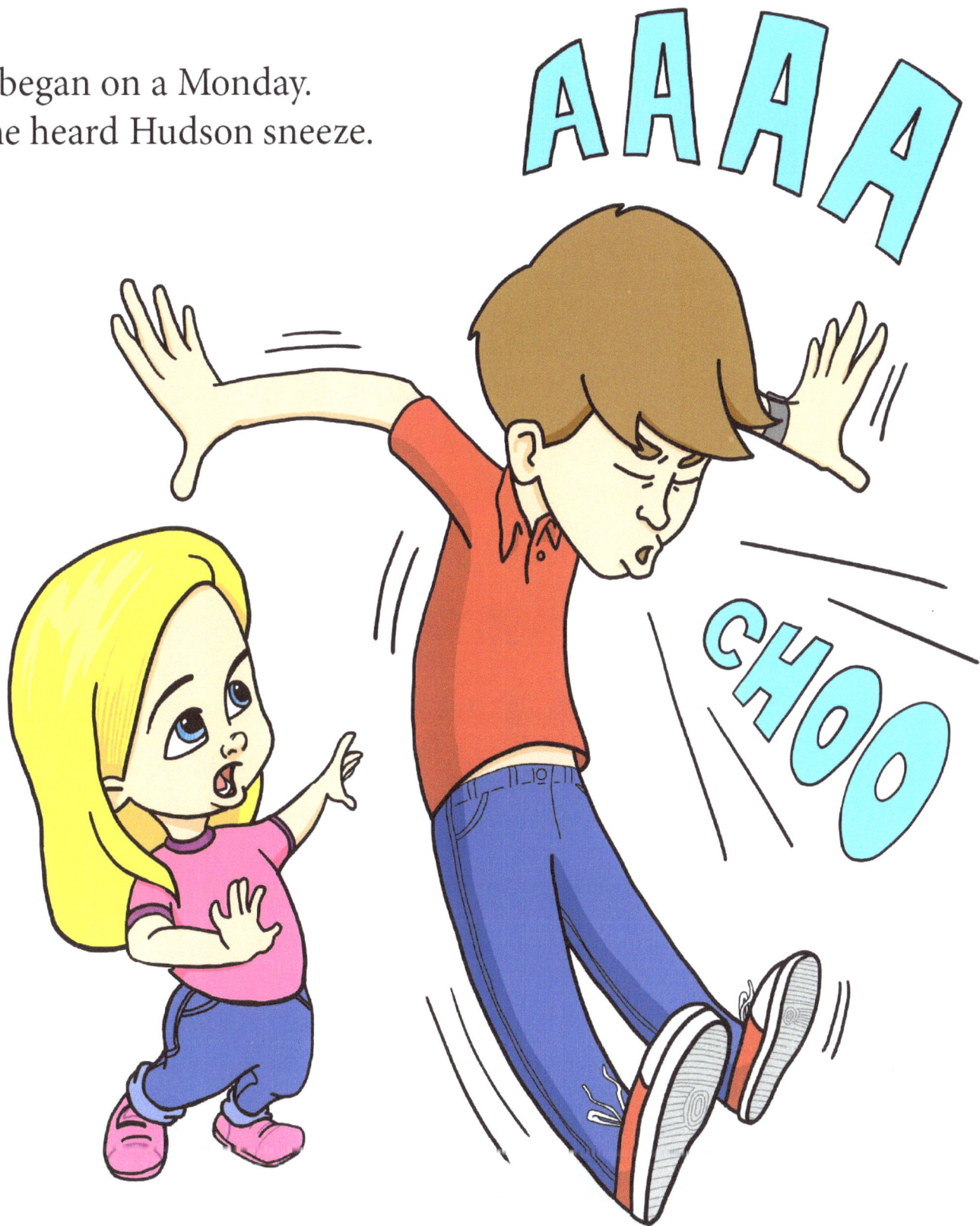

AAAA

CHOO

"My head feels hot. There's a pain in my knees.
My fingers feel funny. I cough when I talk.
There's a buzz in my nose. I feel strange when I walk."

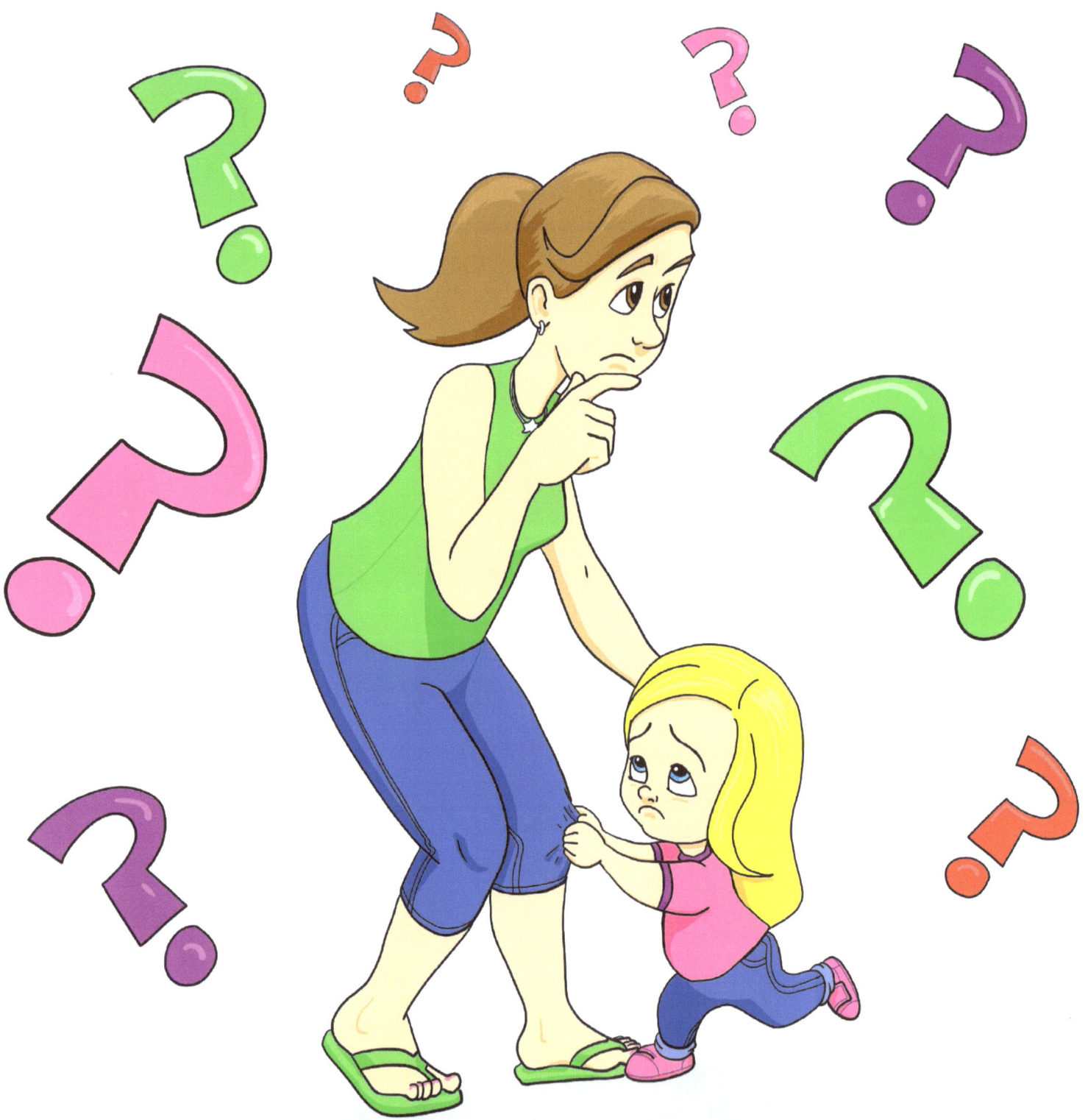

"What's happened to Hudson, Mom? Juliette asked.
"Will he have to miss school? Will you keep him in bed?

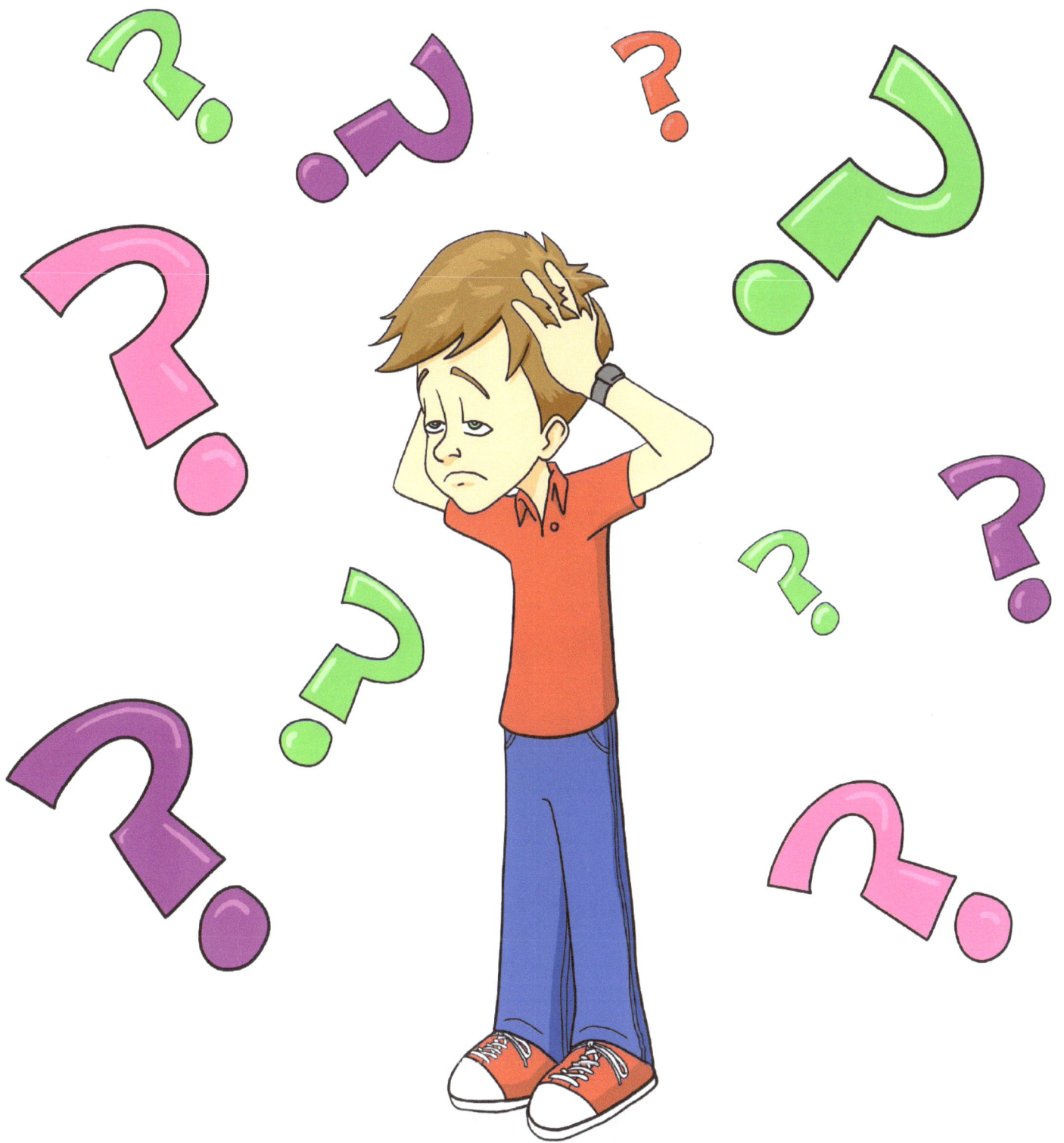

"What makes people sick?
Do you have some suggestions?
When someone feels bad,
there are so many questions!"

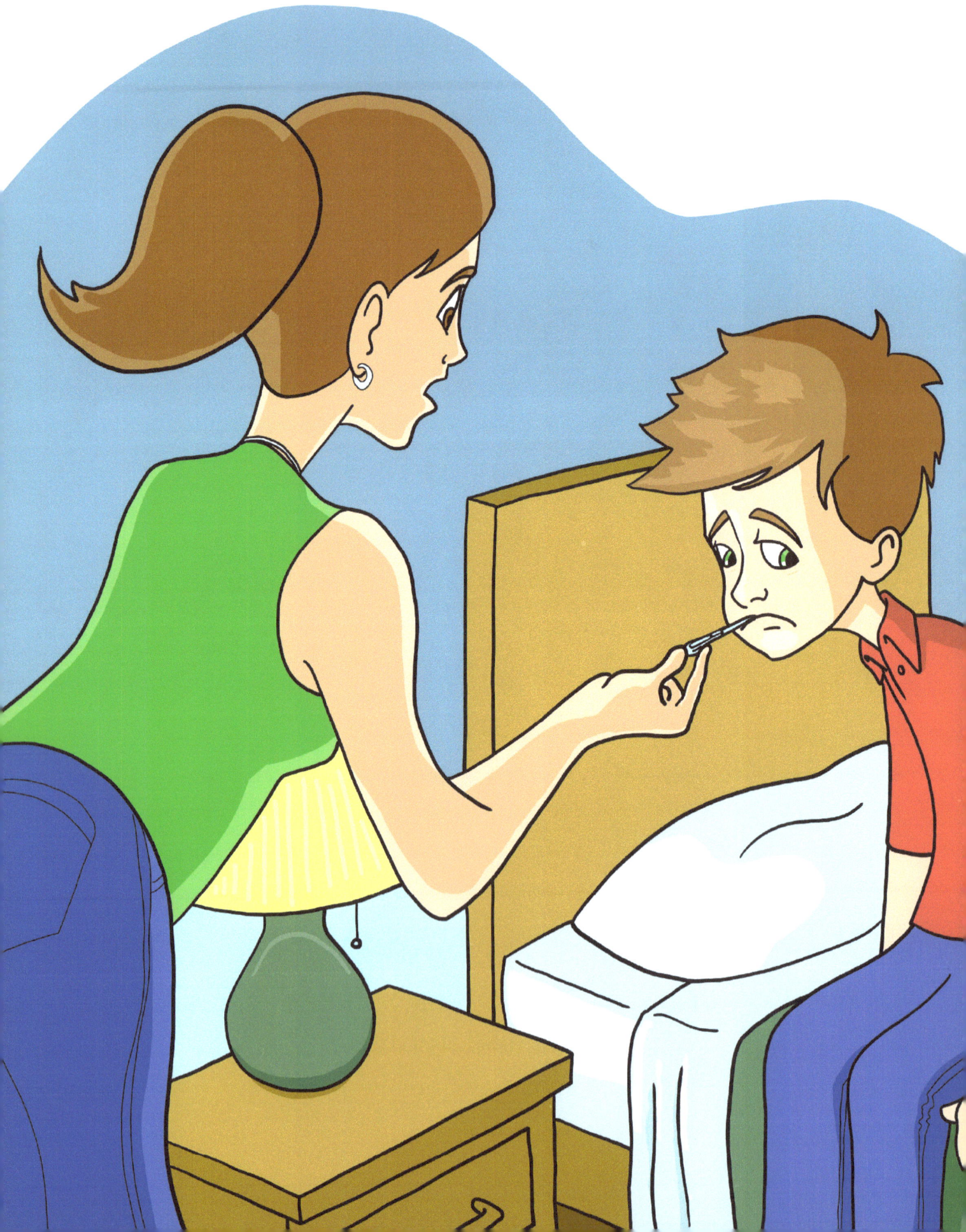

Juliette's mom knew just what to do.
She took Hudson's temperature. One-hundred point two!
"We'll go to the doctor," said Juliette's mother,
"to discover the bug that is bugging your brother."

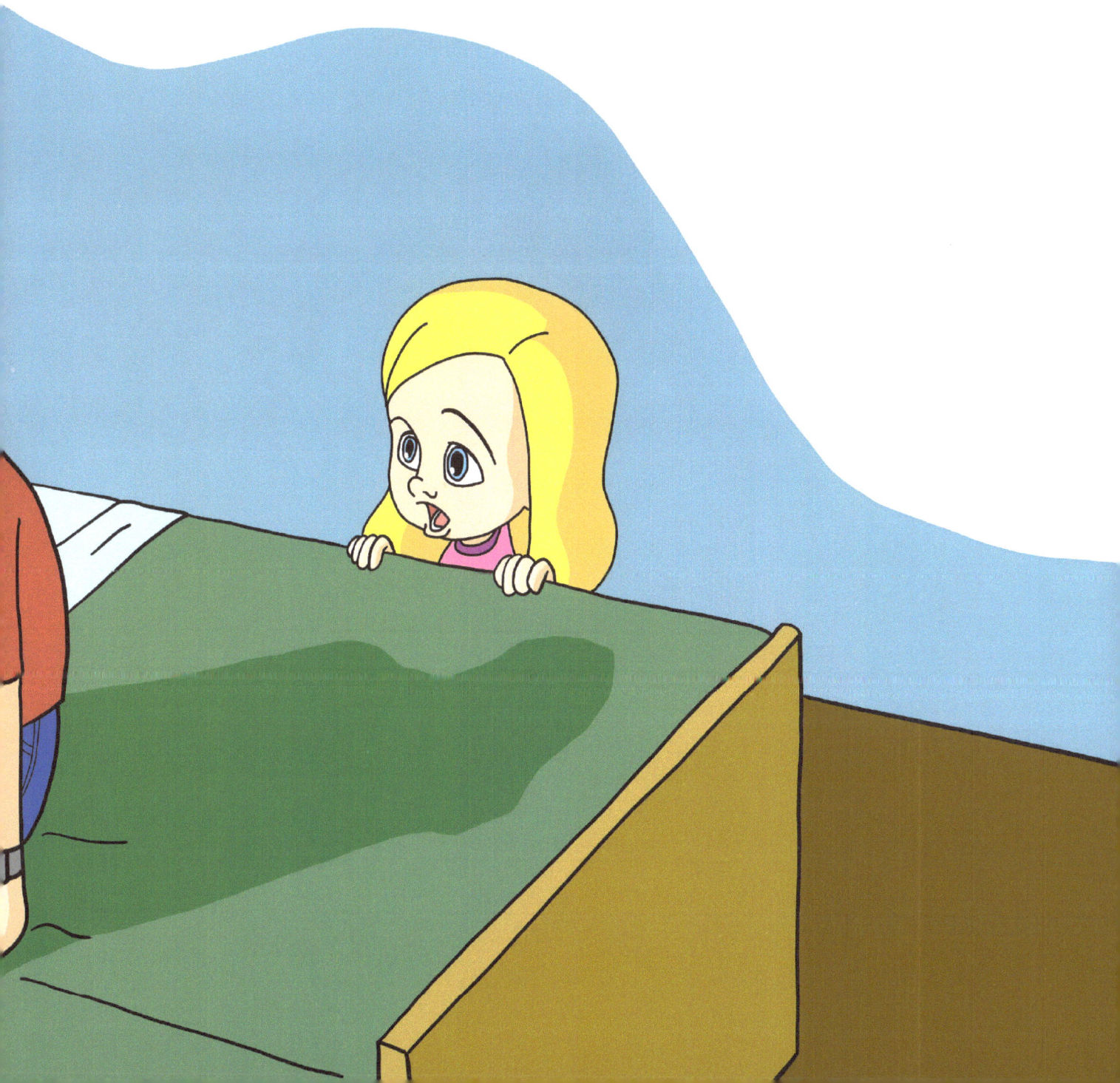

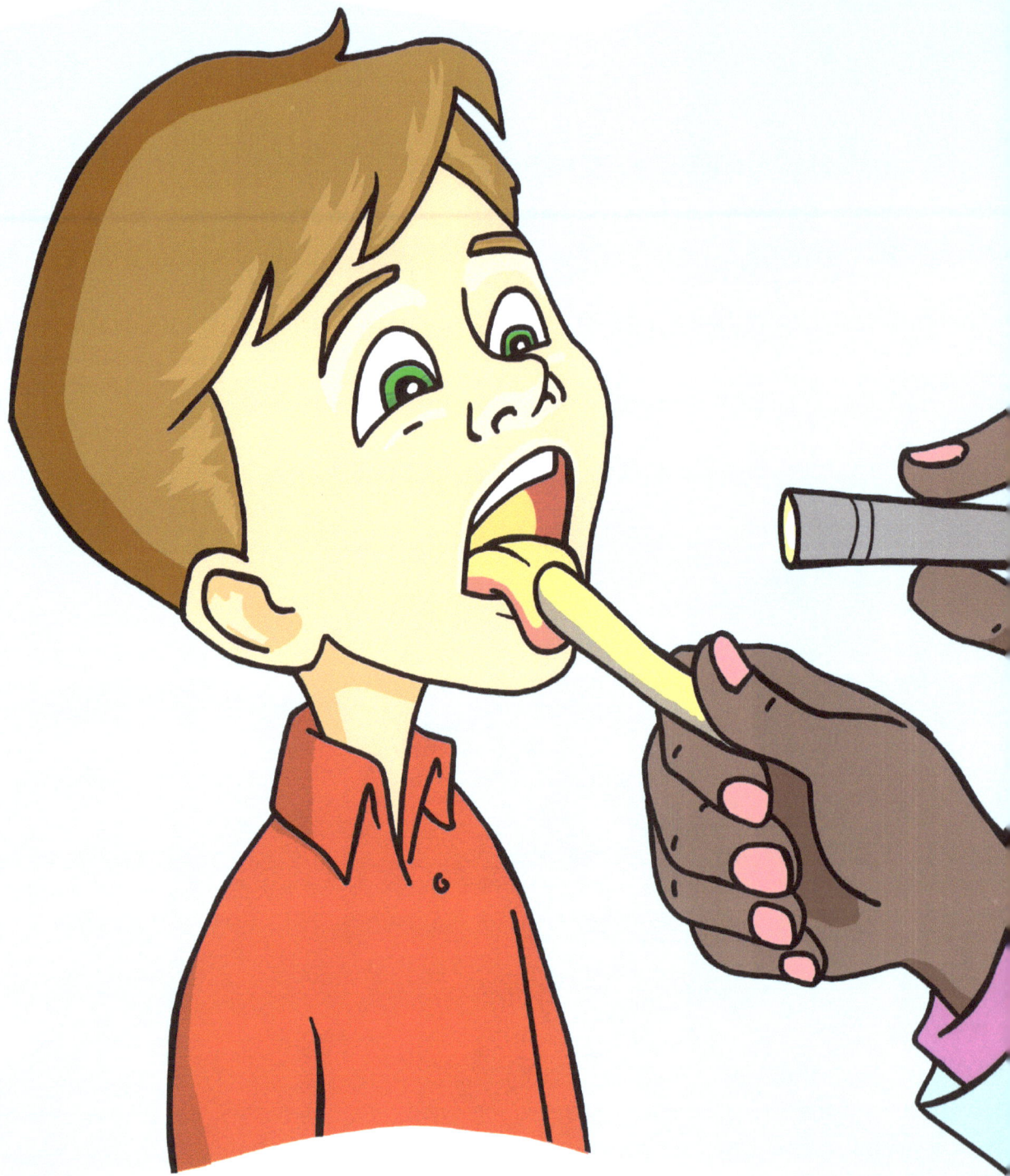

"I'm sorry you're achy," the good doctor said.
She asked where it hurt, and she felt Hudson's head.
She probed Hudson's ears with a shiny white light,
examined his throat and said, "Something's not right."
She swabbed Hudson's tongue, saying, "This is a test.
Until we know more, please get plenty of rest.
Take these pills for your fever, and drink lots of water."

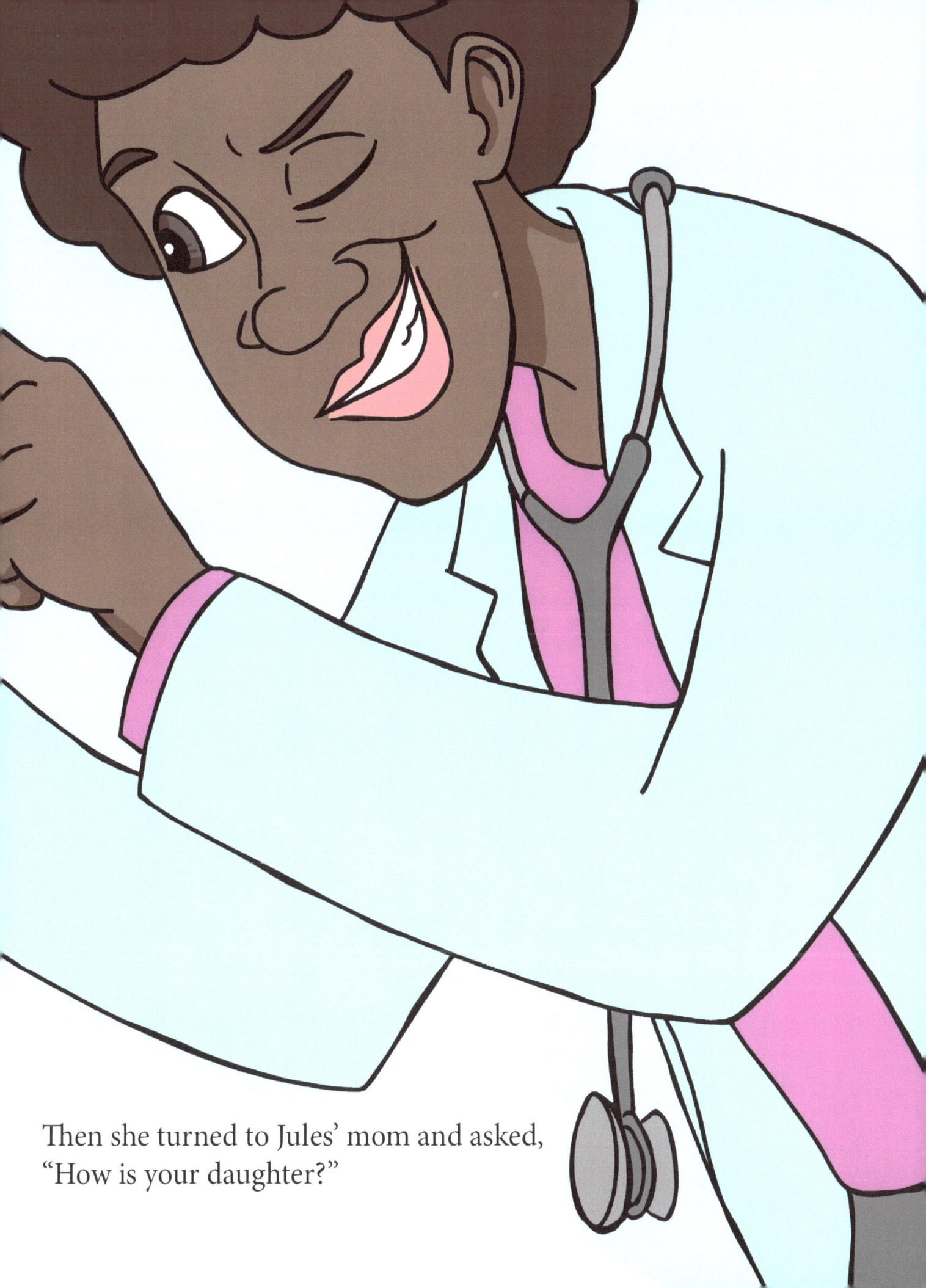

Then she turned to Jules' mom and asked,
"How is your daughter?"

Juliette answered, "I feel fine today.
How can I make Hudson's bug go away?"

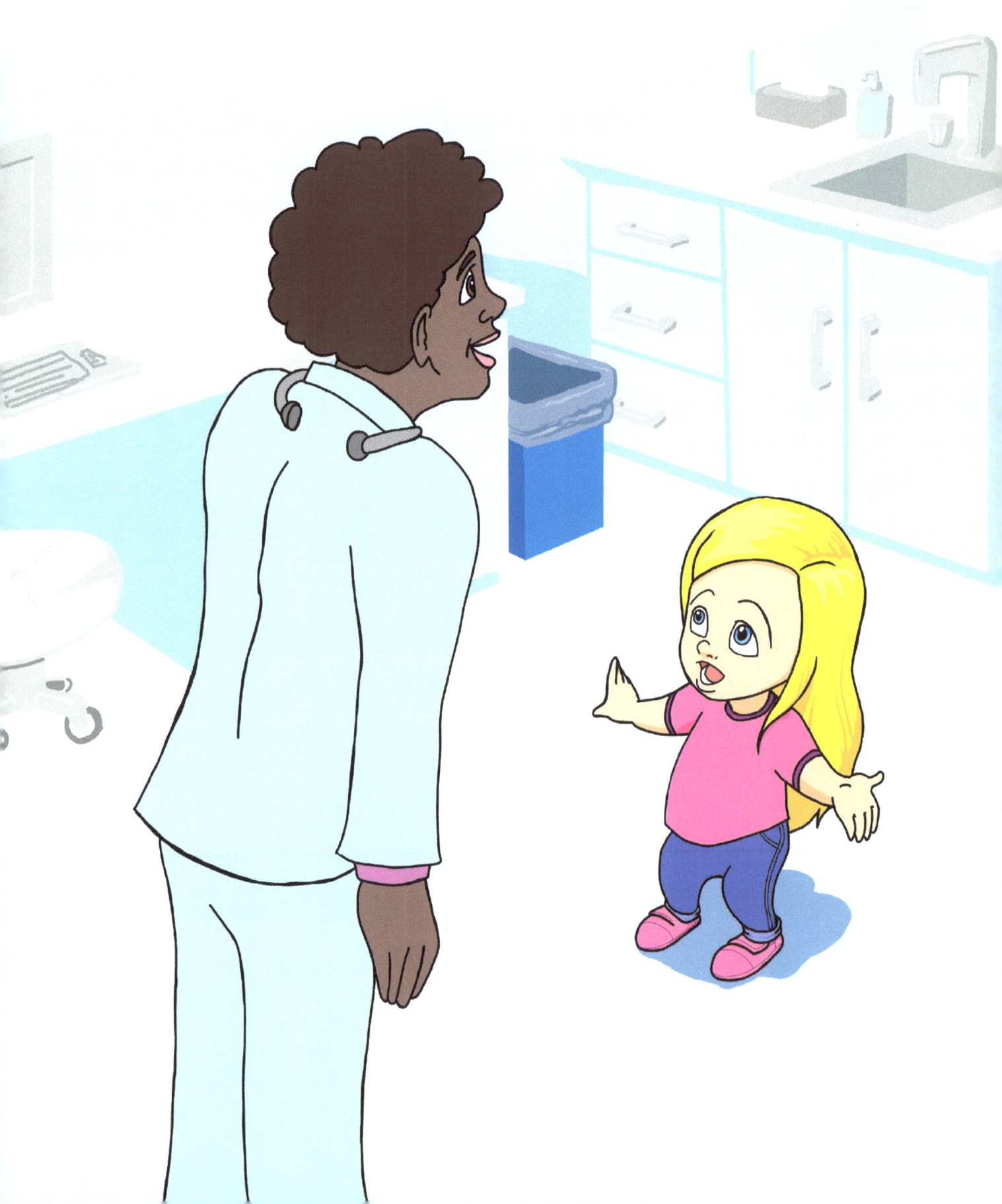

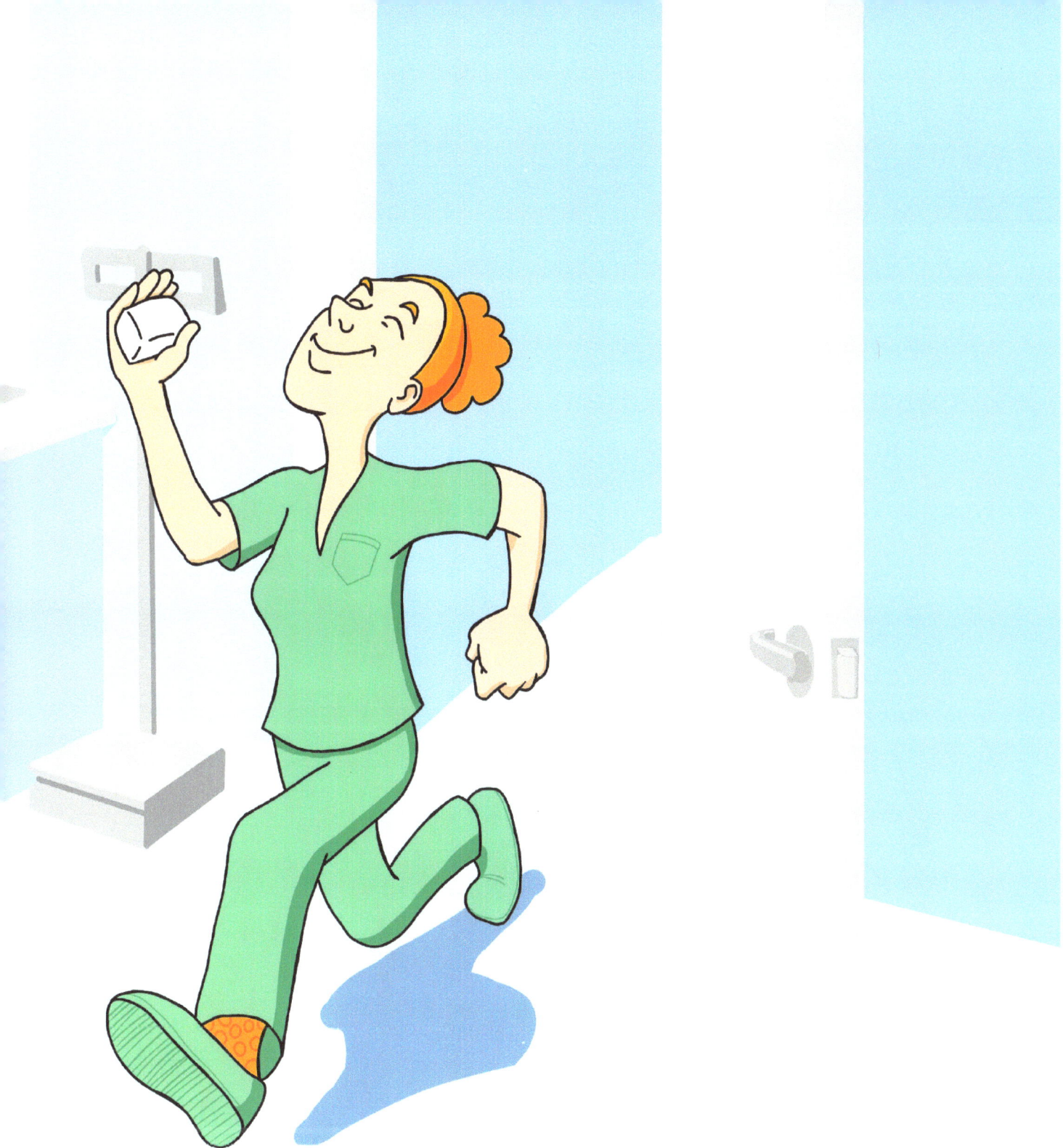

"I'll have my nurse teach some things you can do
to stomp out the bugs that cause colds and flu."
Then in came the nurse, Ms. Veronica Sands.
She held out some soap and said, "Let's wash our hands."

"We wash before breakfast,
we wash before lunch,
we wash before dinner,
we wash when we munch.

After basketball, football,
and when we feel snotty.
After playing with puppies...

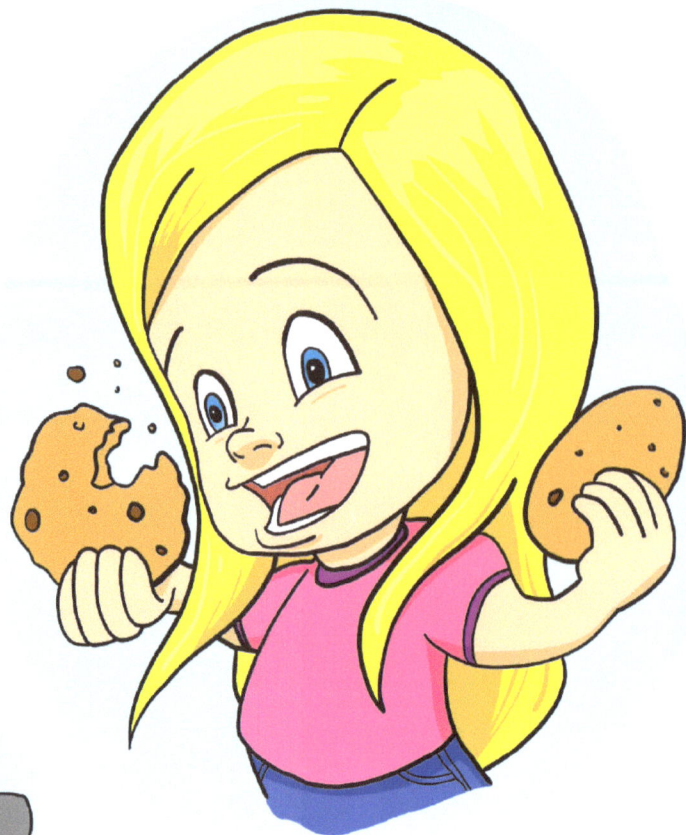

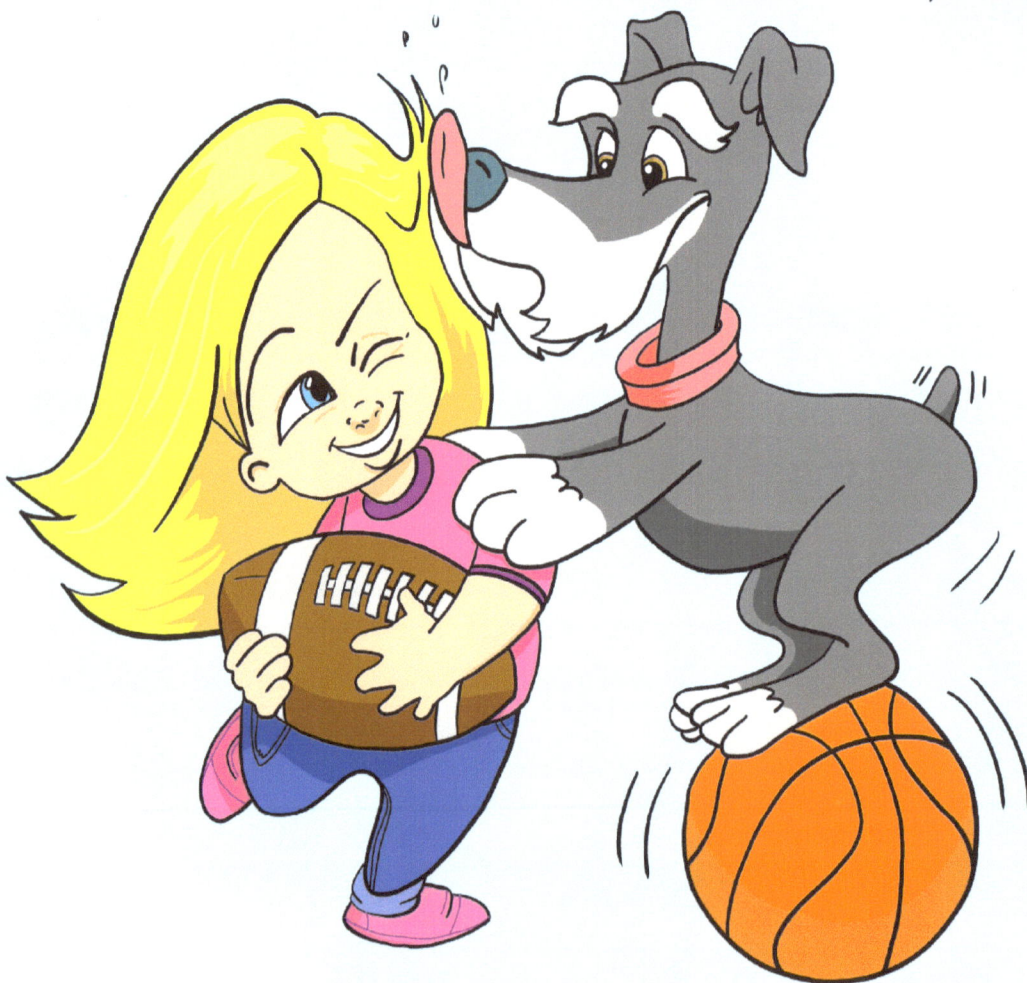

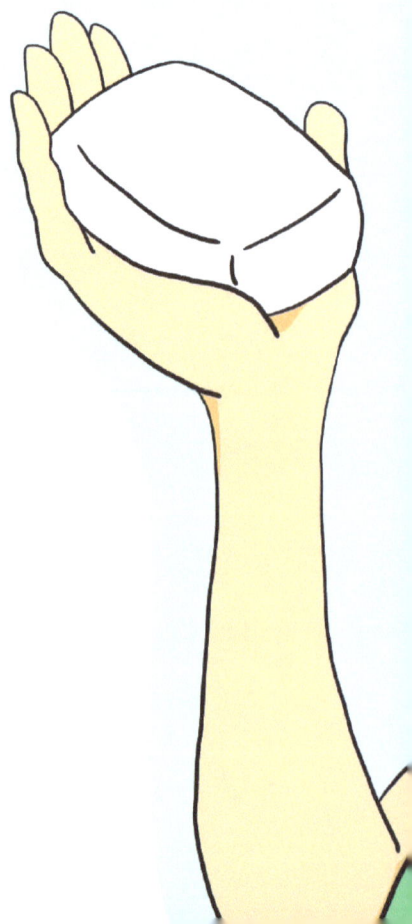

and after we potty."

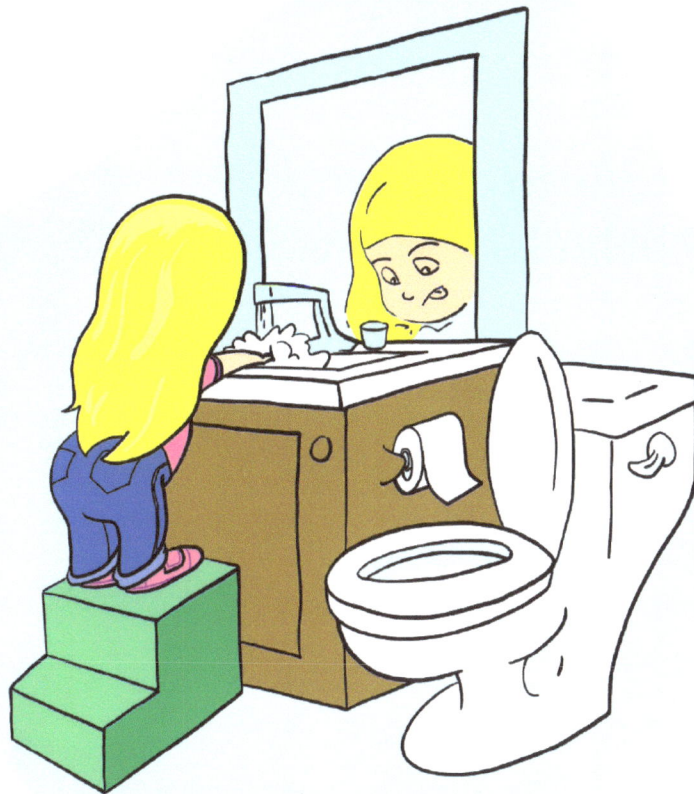

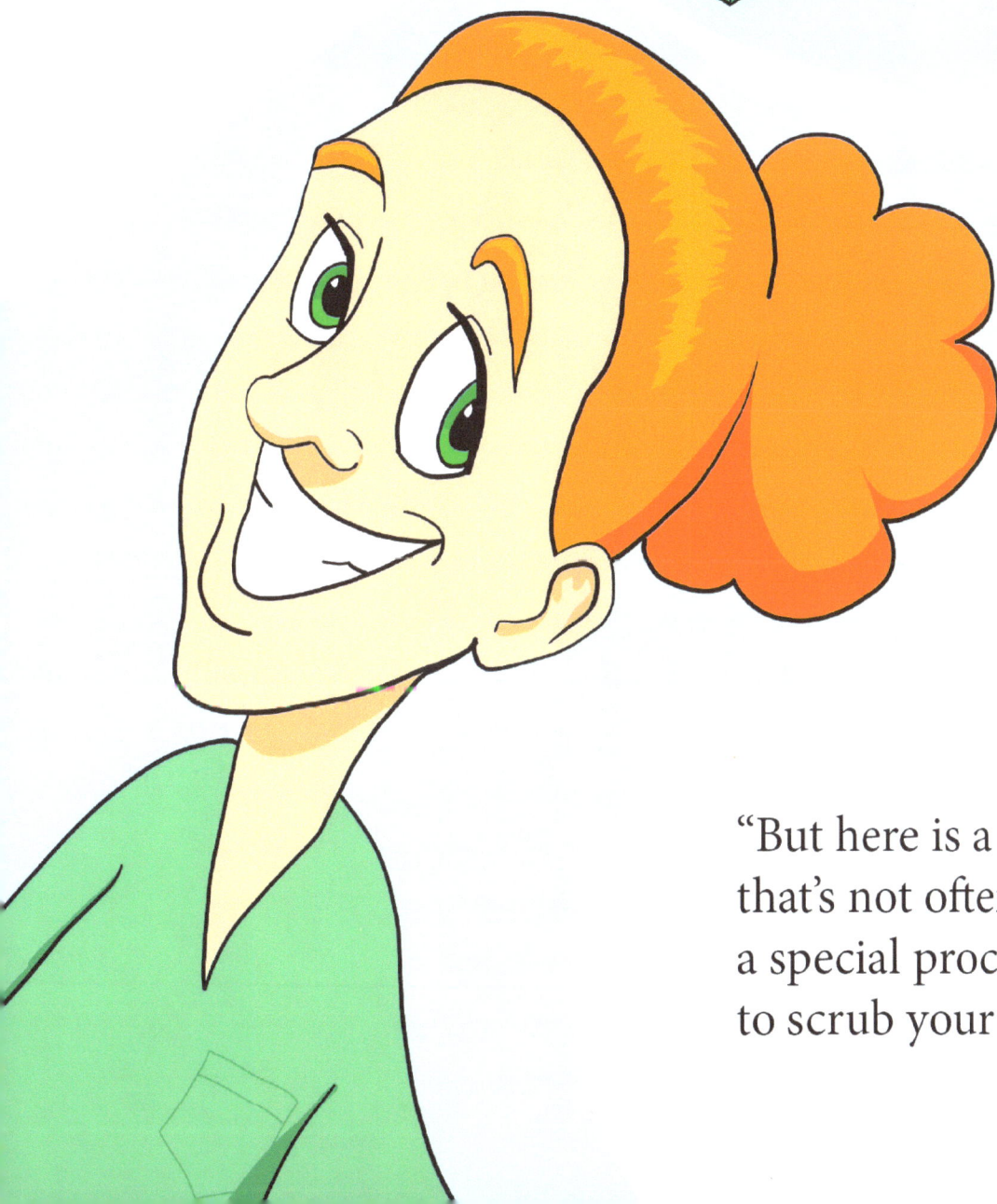

"But here is a secret
that's not often seen,
a special procedure
to scrub your hands clean."

She lathered the soap
until both hands were white

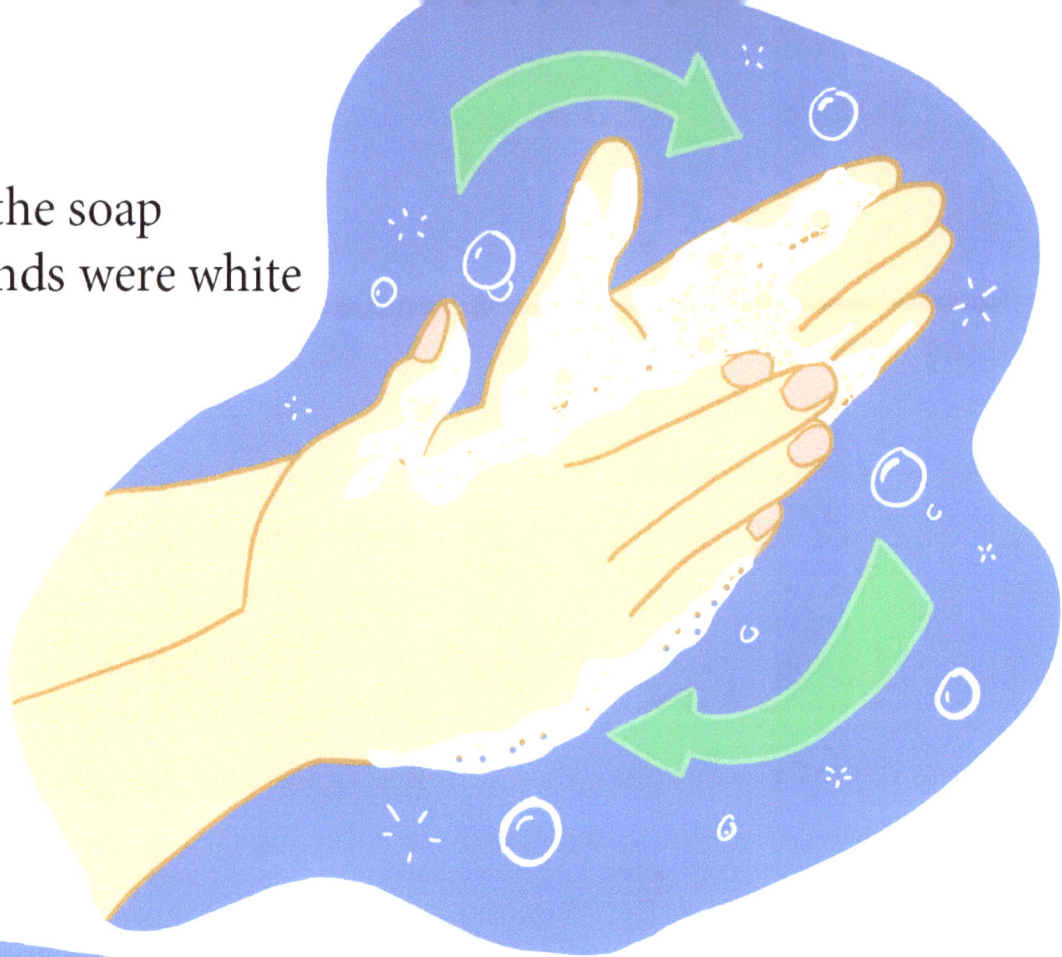

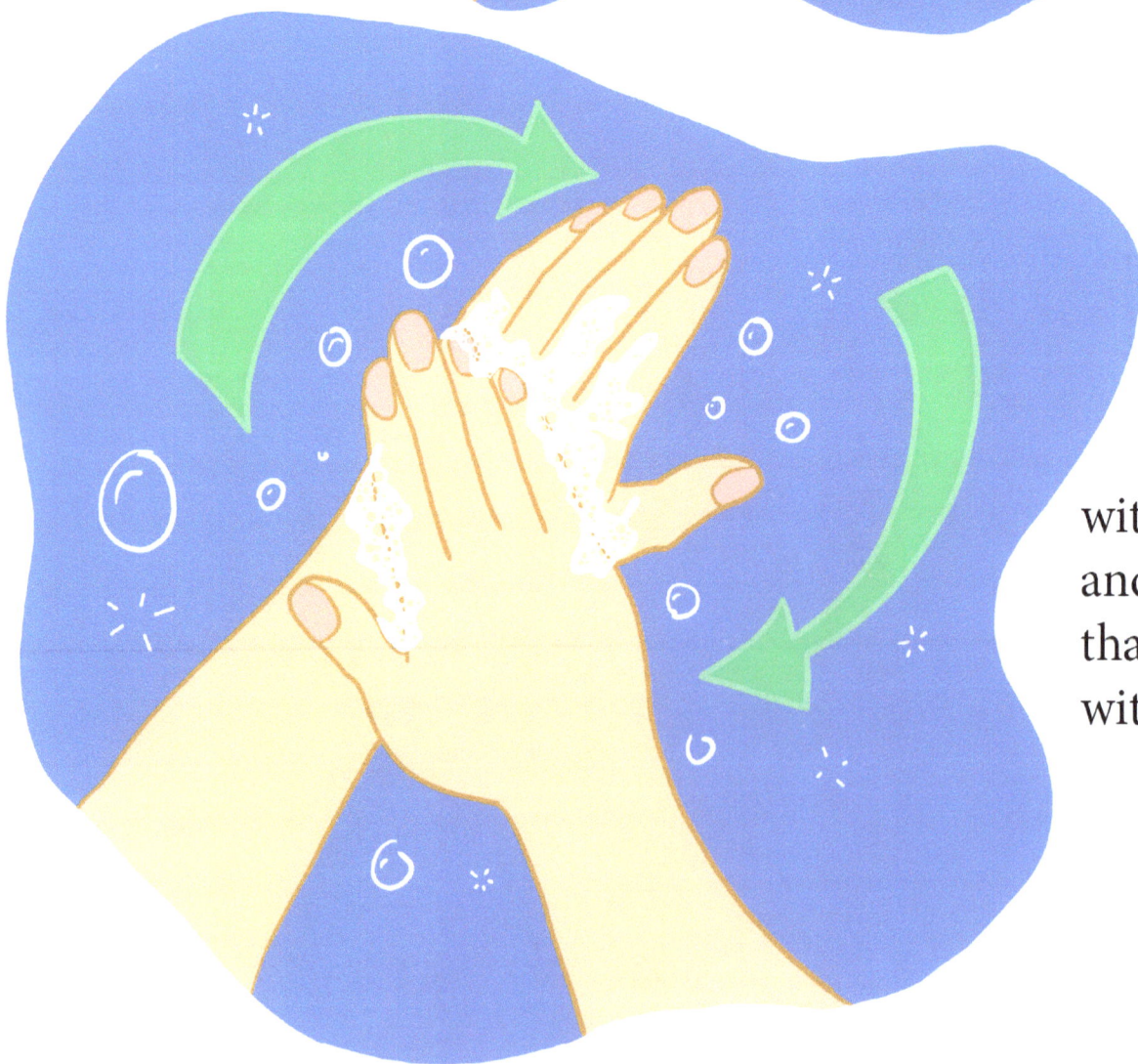

with bubbles
and scrubbles
that popped
with delight.

She scrubbed
every finger,

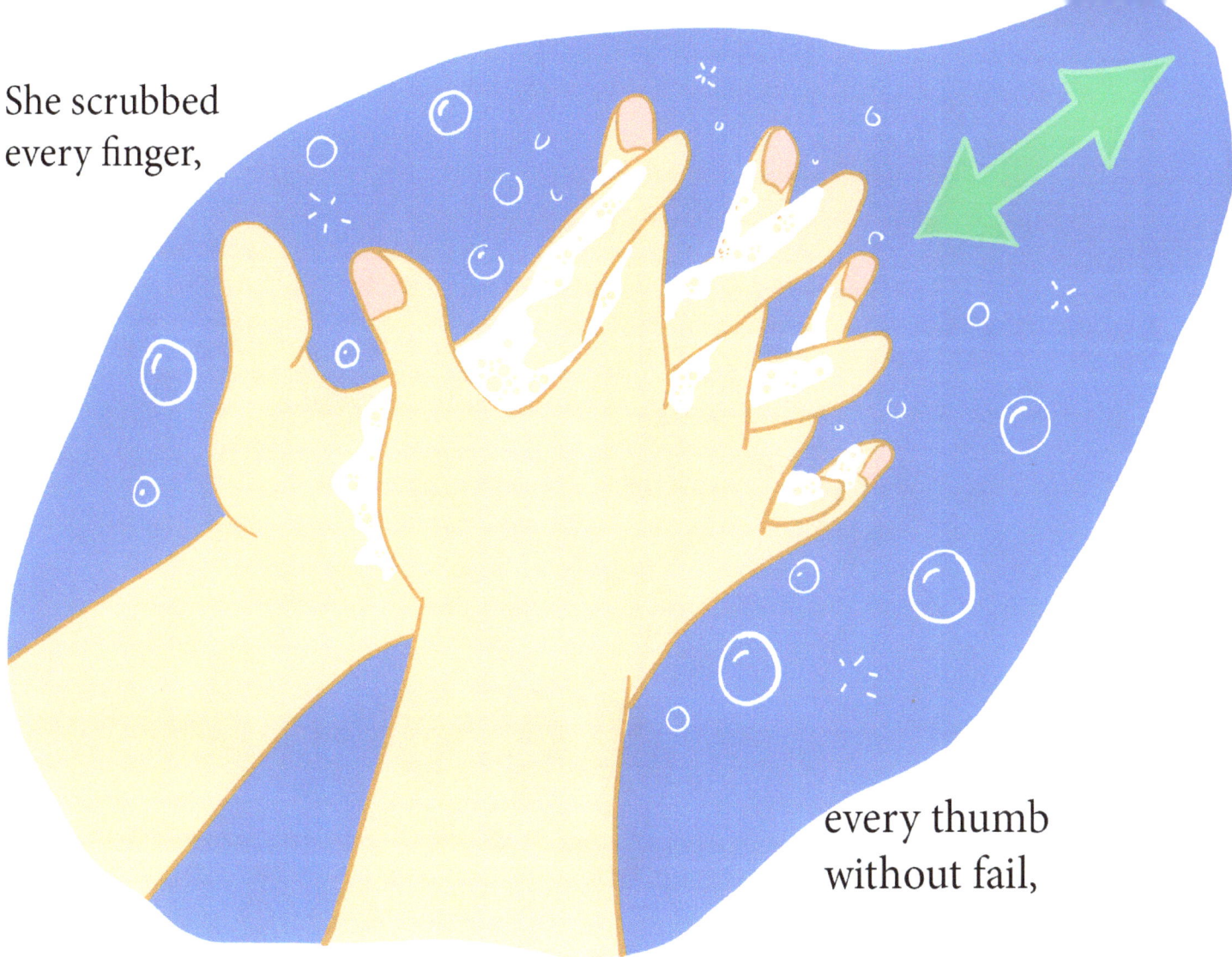

every thumb
without fail,

she dug out
the dirt
from beneath
every nail.

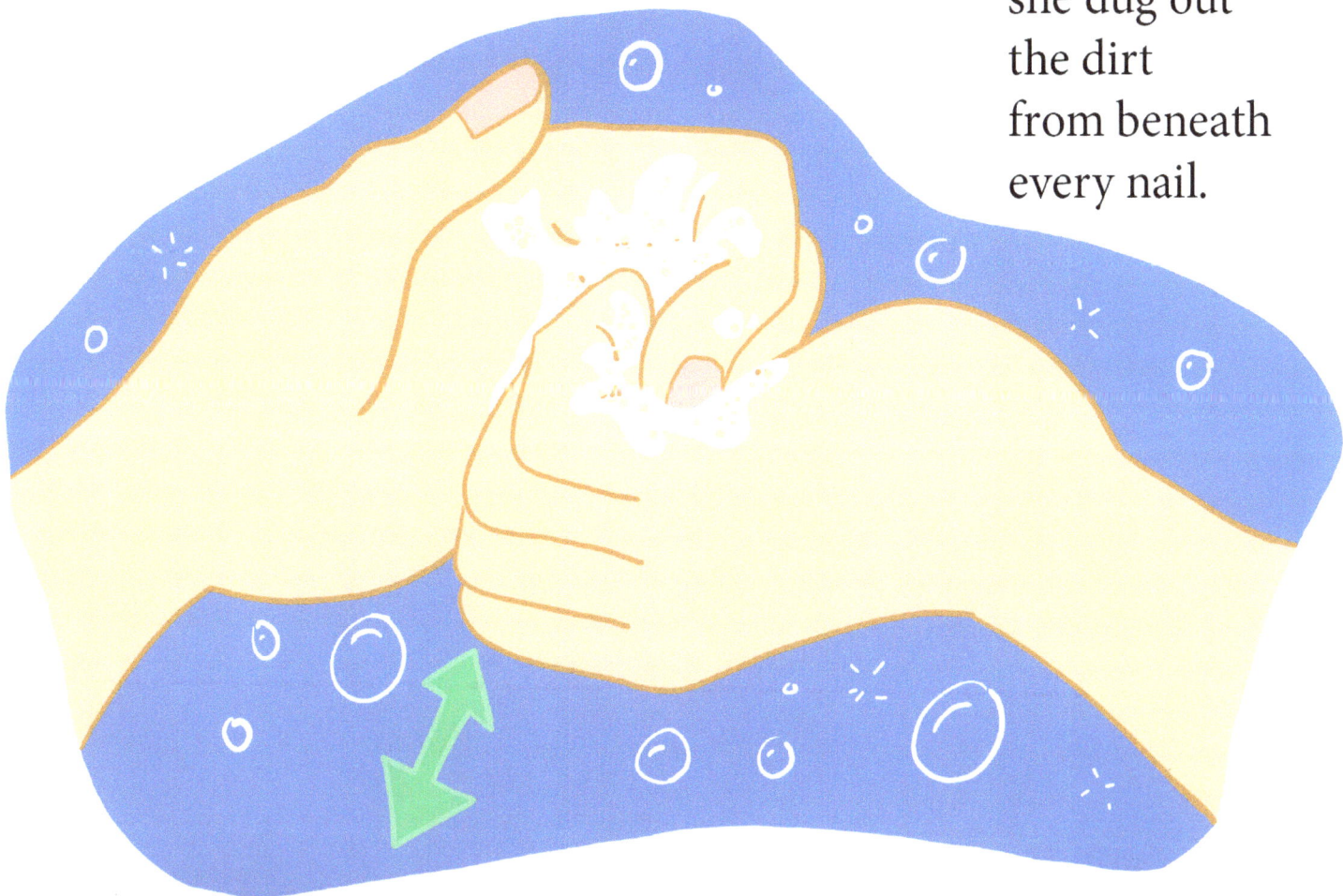

She washed and she scrubbed,
counting twenty from one.
Then she rinsed with warm water,
saying, "Wasn't that fun?"

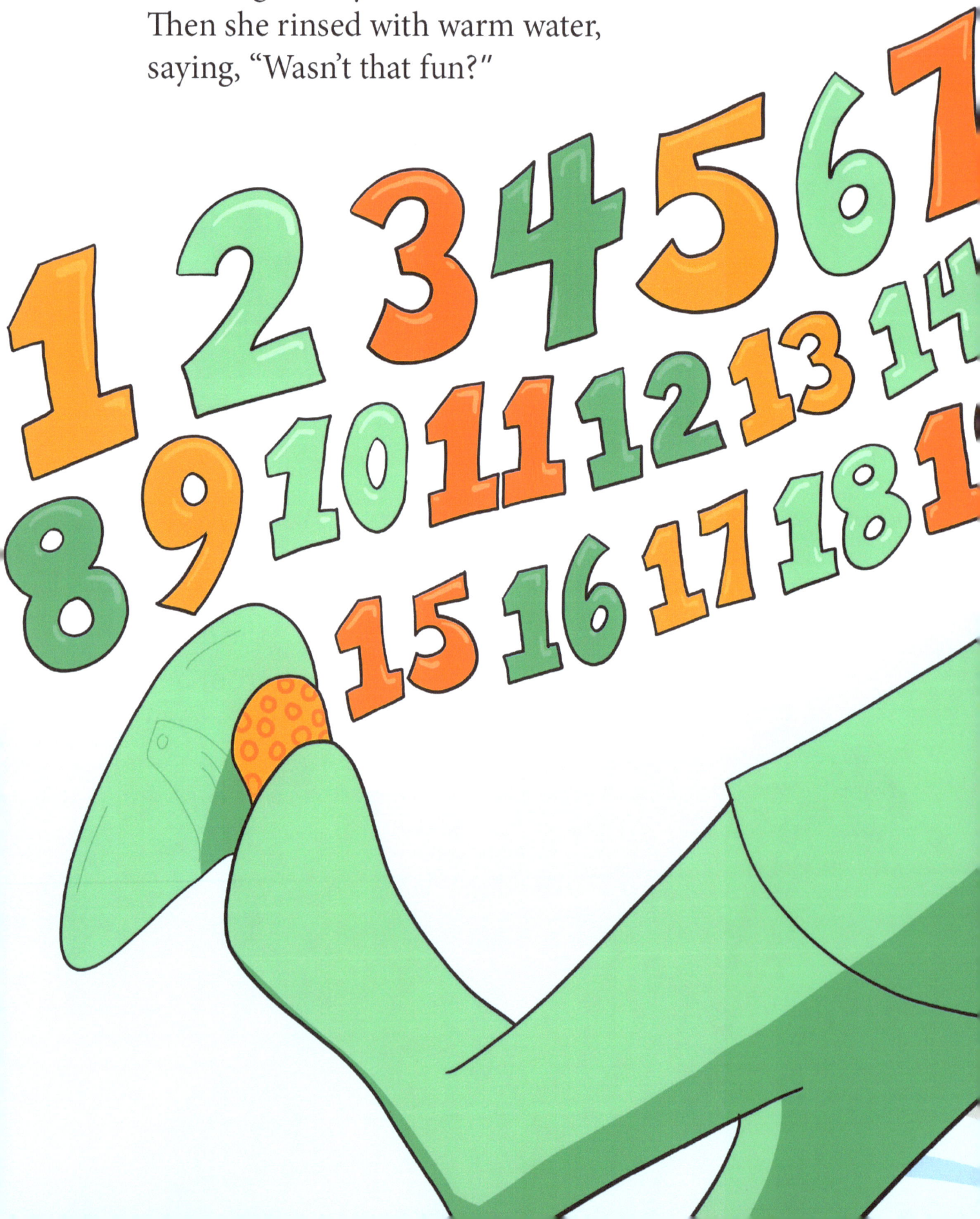

1 2 3 4 5 6 7
8 9 10 11 12 13 14
15 16 17 18 1

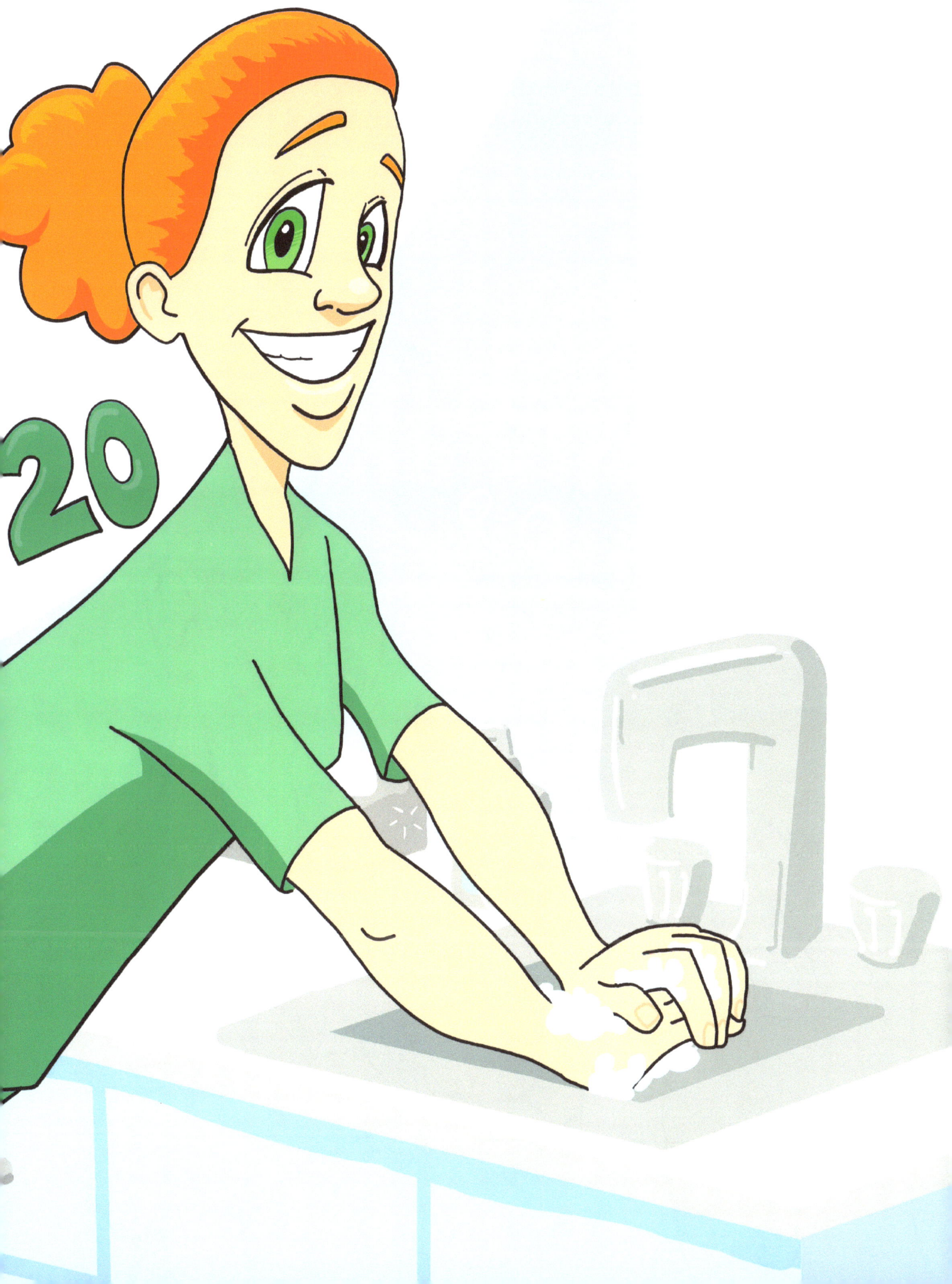

"That took a long time," Hudson said in surprise.
"Some germs," the nurse said, "you can't see with your eyes.
Warm water and scrubbing will get the job done,
and once you know how, it is really quite fun."

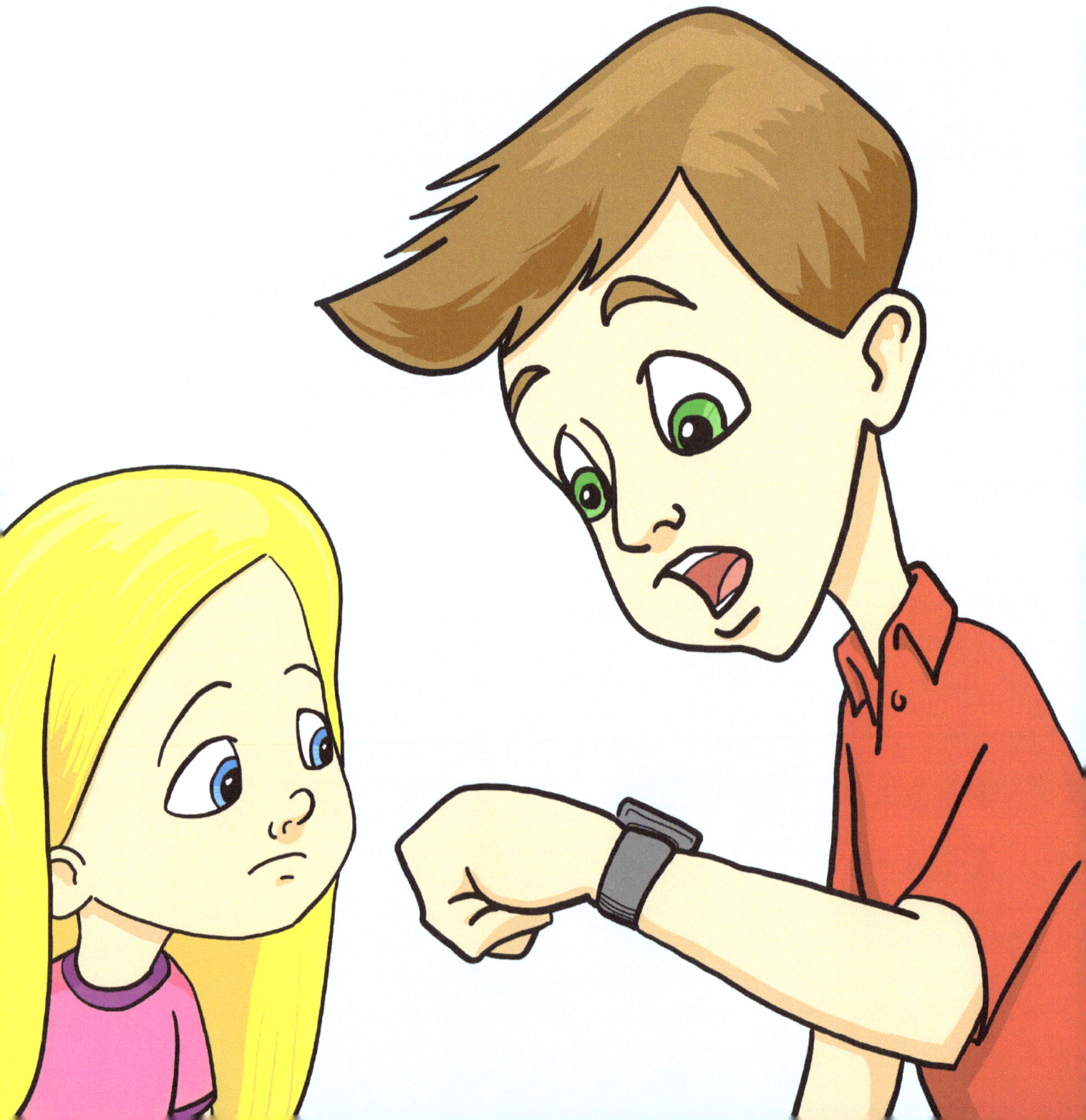

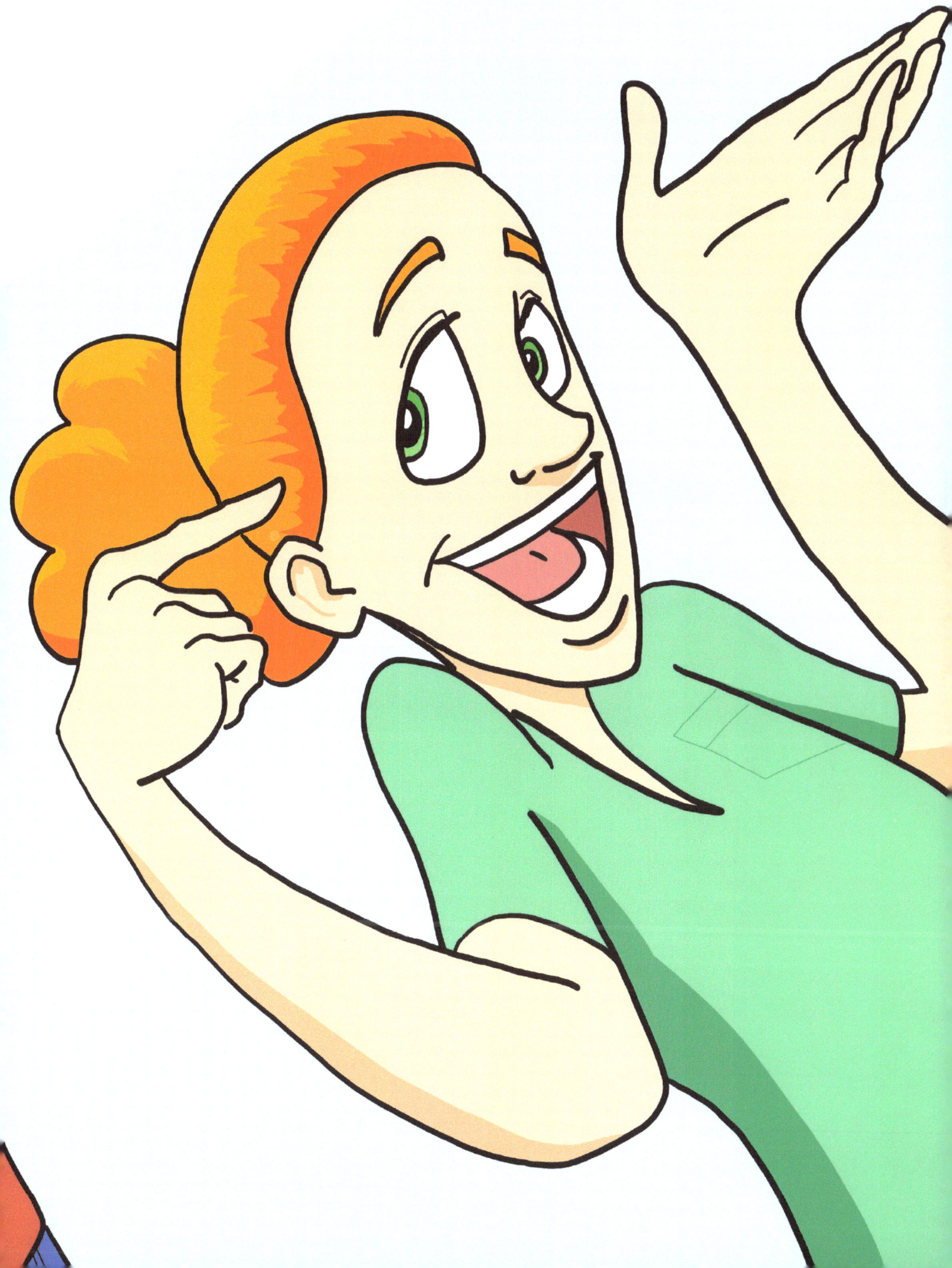

Jules exclaimed with delight, "Tell us more! Tell us more!
How do we push all those germs out the door?
"I'll teach you a trick," said the nurse. "It's a breeze.
It's a thing you can do whenever you sneeze.

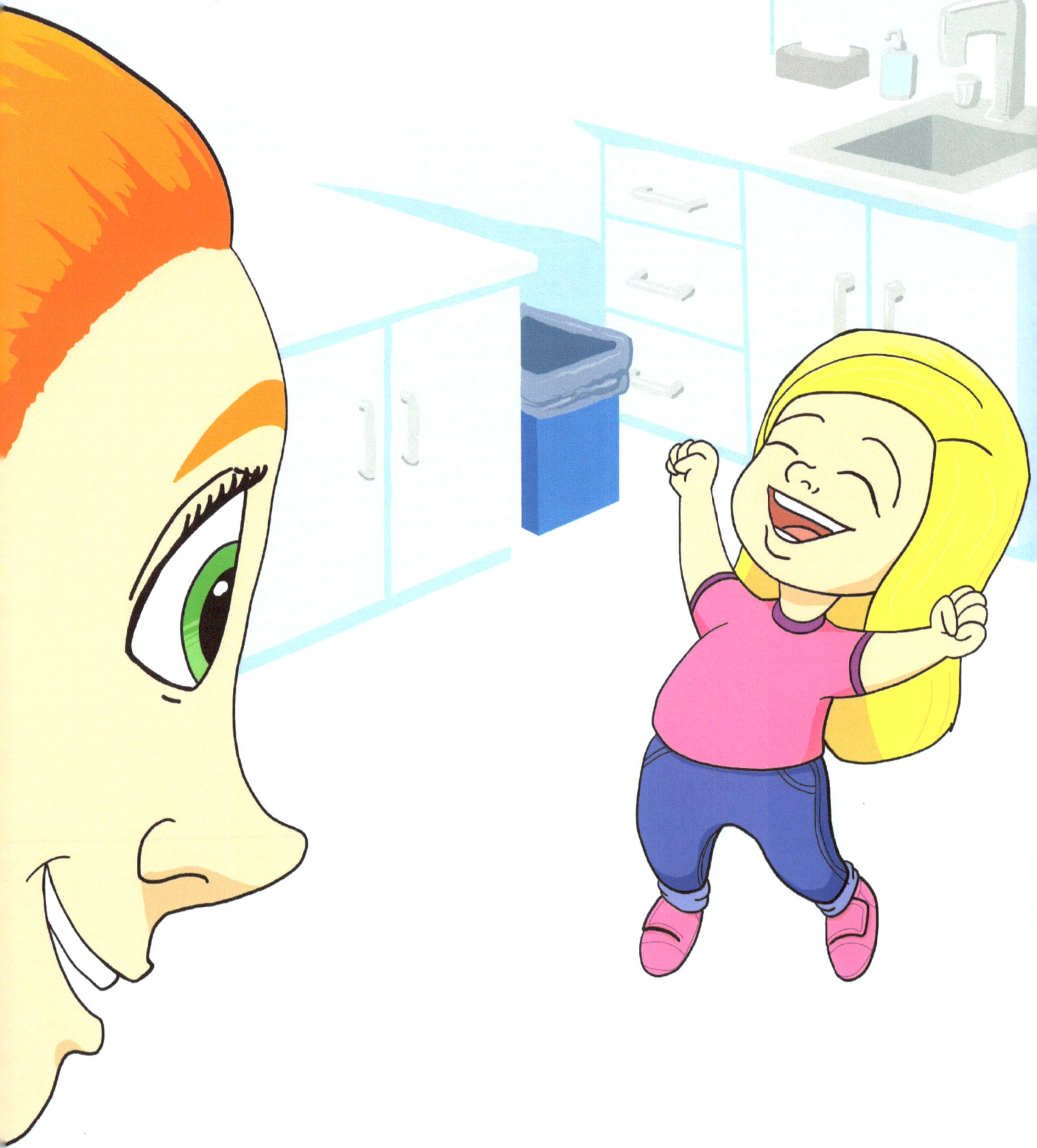

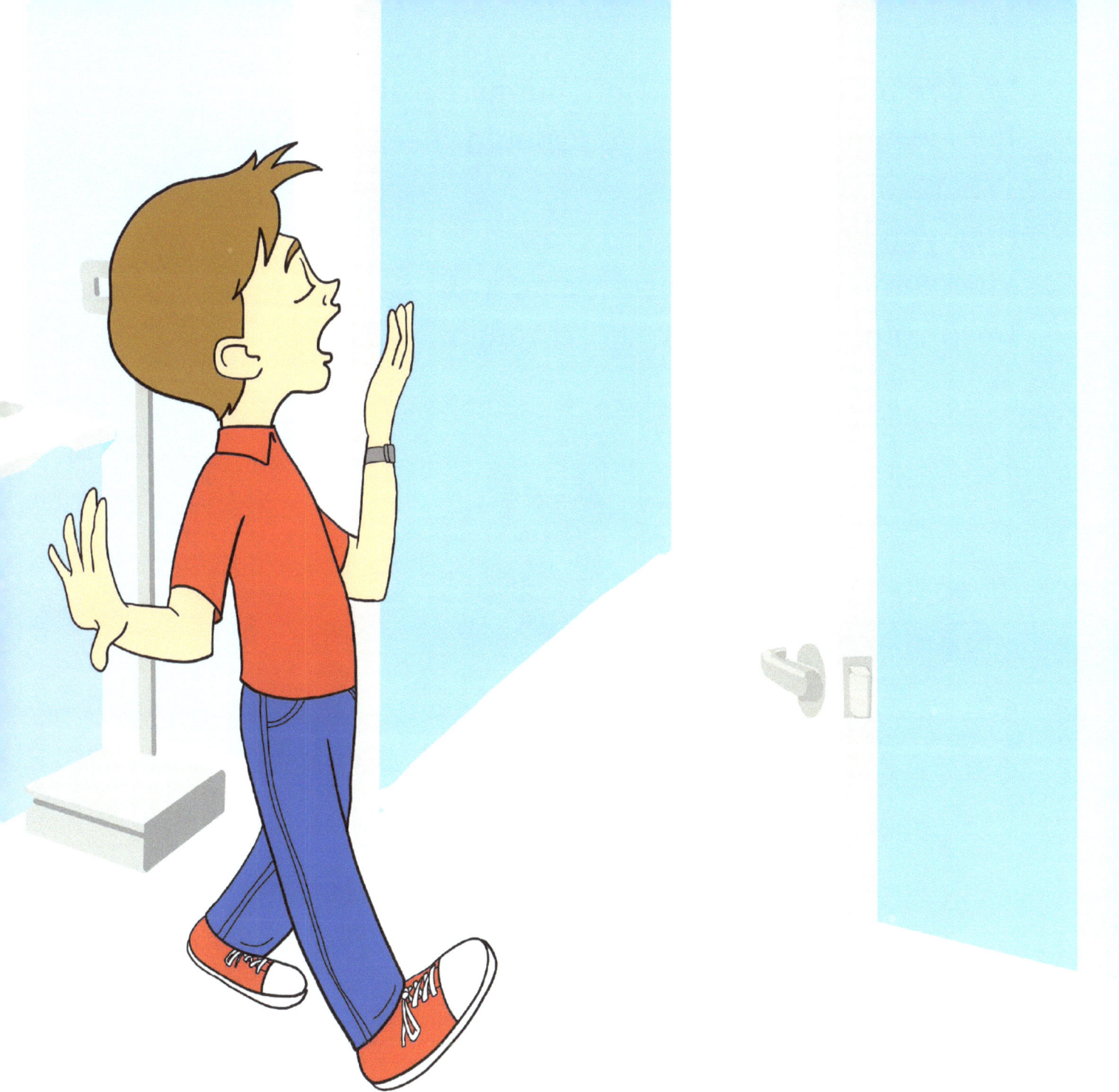

"I know how to sneeze," Hudson said with a yawn.
"If you cover your mouth, you won't pass the bugs on."

"You're partly right. Hudson, but here is the issue:
If you want to trap bugs, you should sneeze in a tissue.
When you throw it away,
then you know what to do.
Find some soap and warm water,
wash your hands, and you're through!"

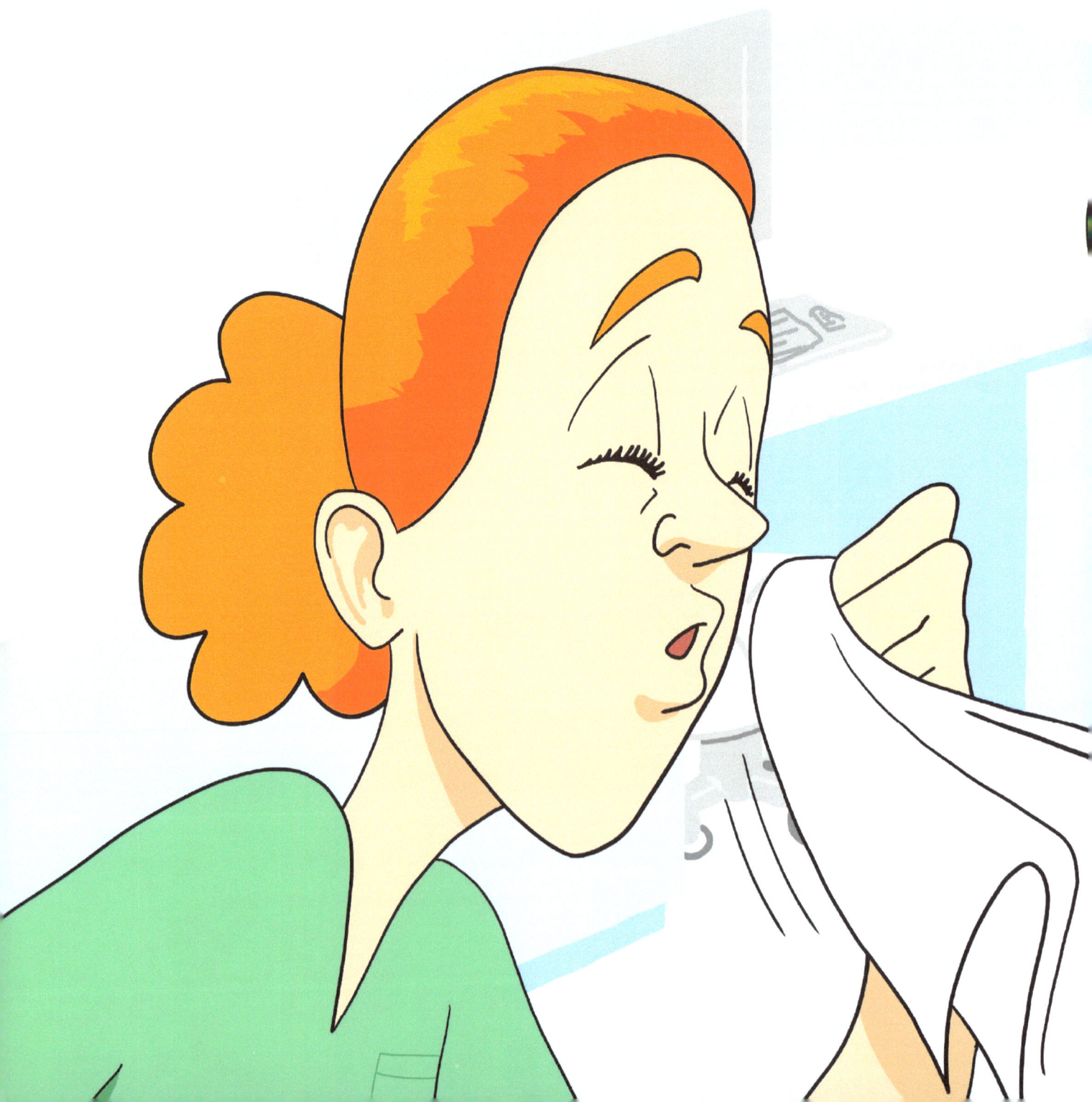

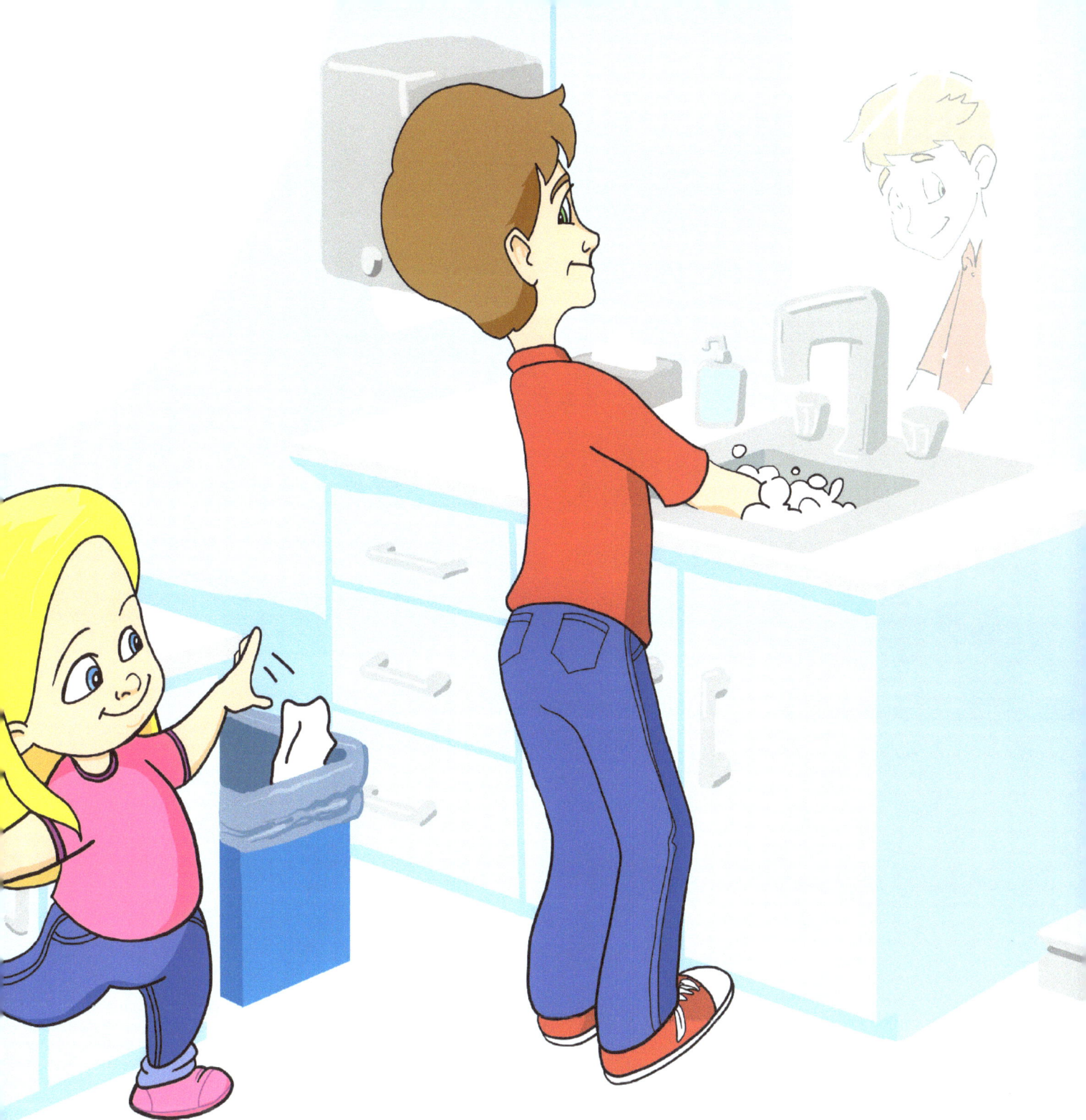

"Now give yourself time,"
said the nurse with a grin.
"Your body can fight this.
Your body can win."

Hudson went home to his bed
quite courageous.
He stayed home from school
while his bug was contagious.

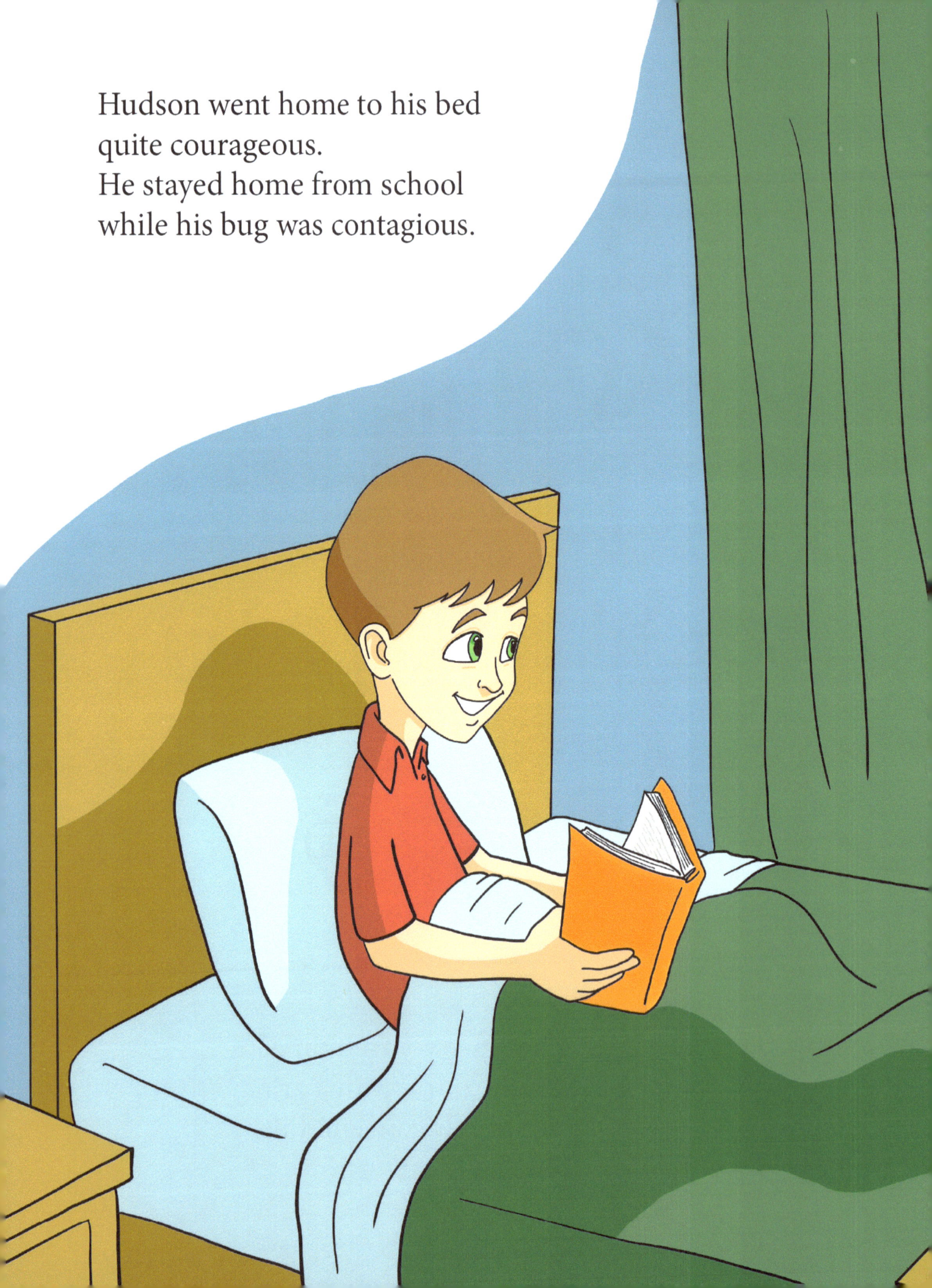

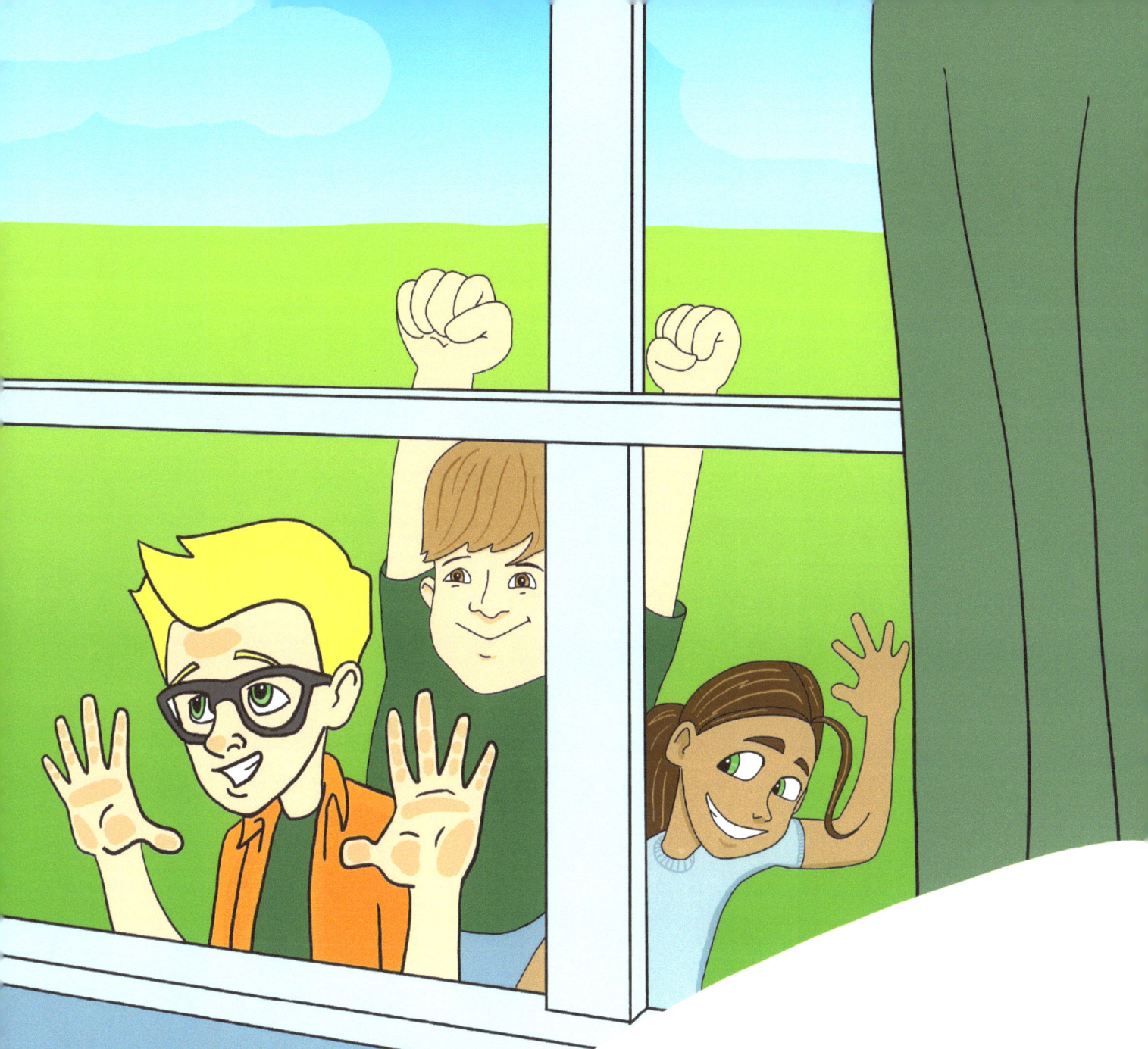

"Contagious" Jules knew
meant that others could catch it,
like Maddux and Asher
and Molly McPatchet.
His teacher, Miss Baggs,
and his basketball friends.
When a person's contagious,
you wait till it ends.

And even though hand washing took a bit longer,
Hudson's nose stopped its running, his muscles felt stronger.
His fever was gone, he could hear, he could smell.
He said to his mother, "I think I am well!"

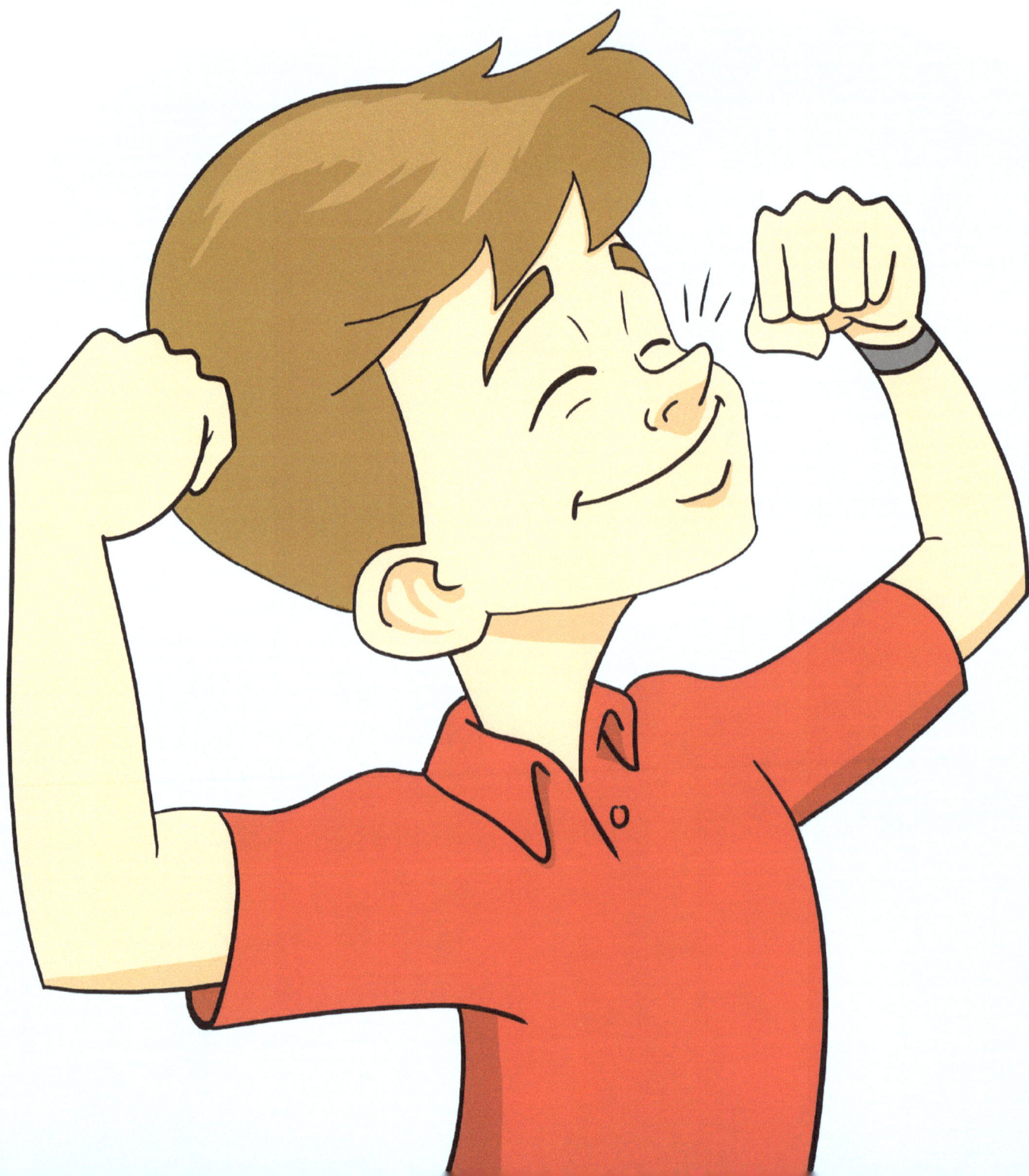

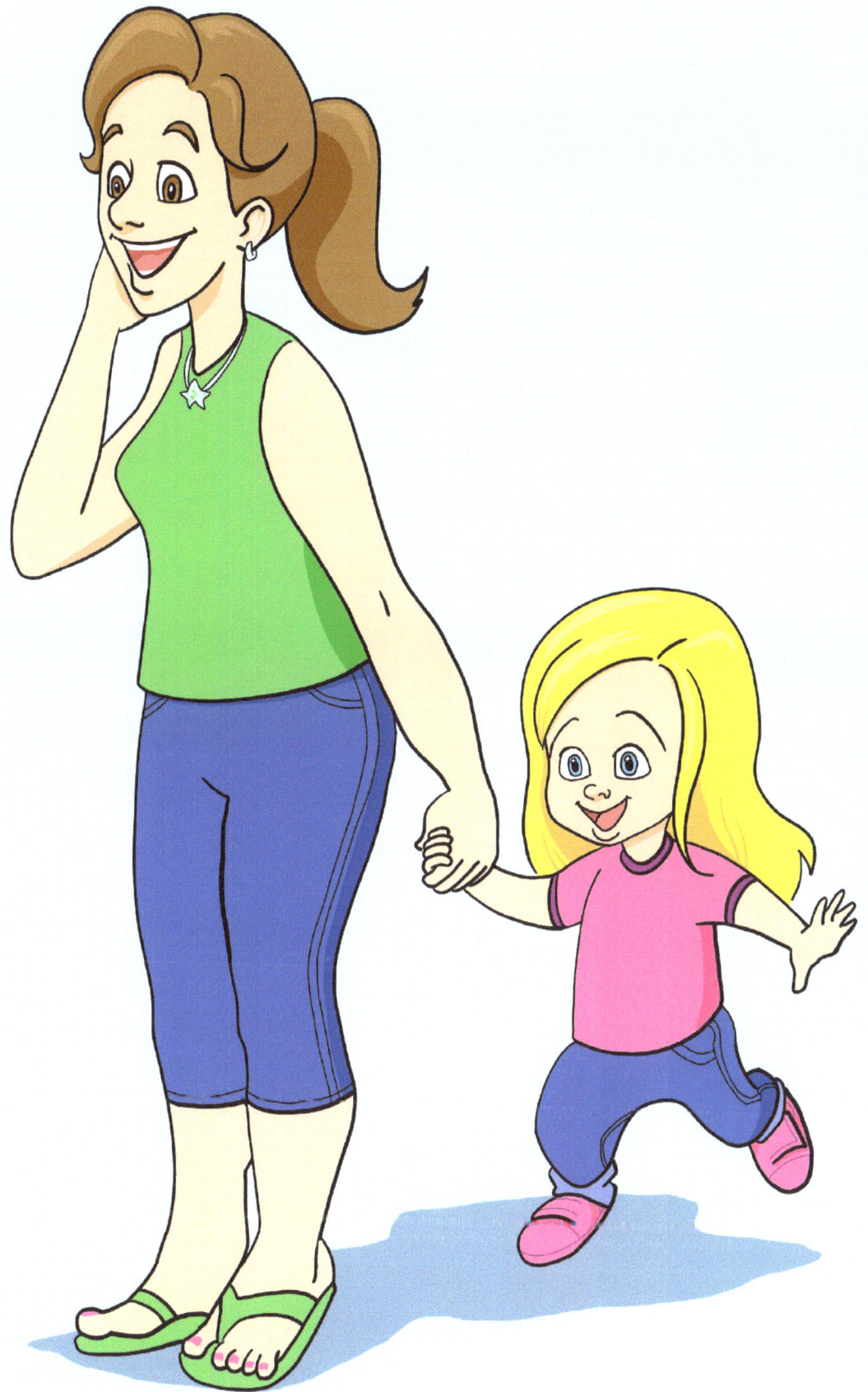

The doctor confirmed. "Hudson's bug went away."

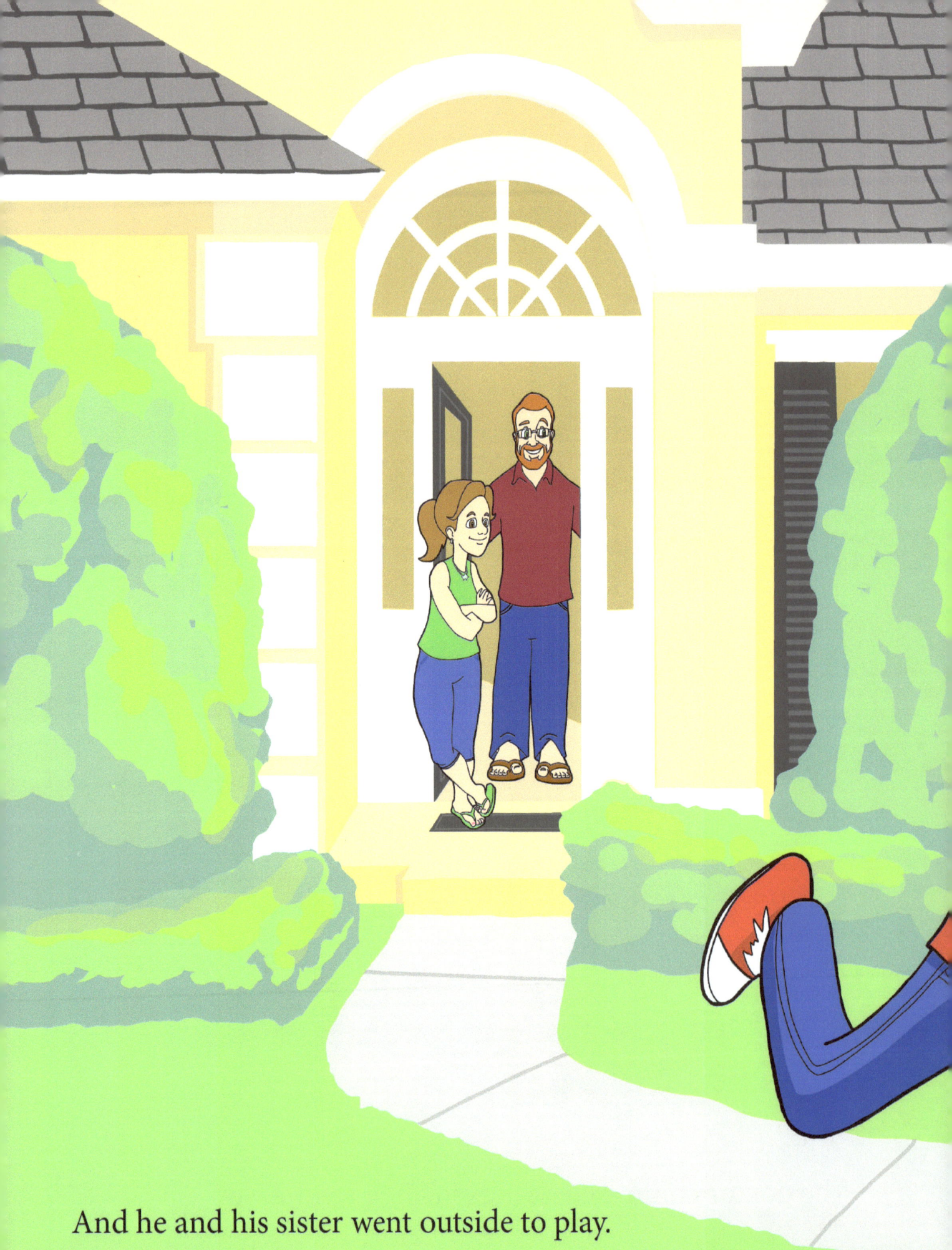

And he and his sister went outside to play.

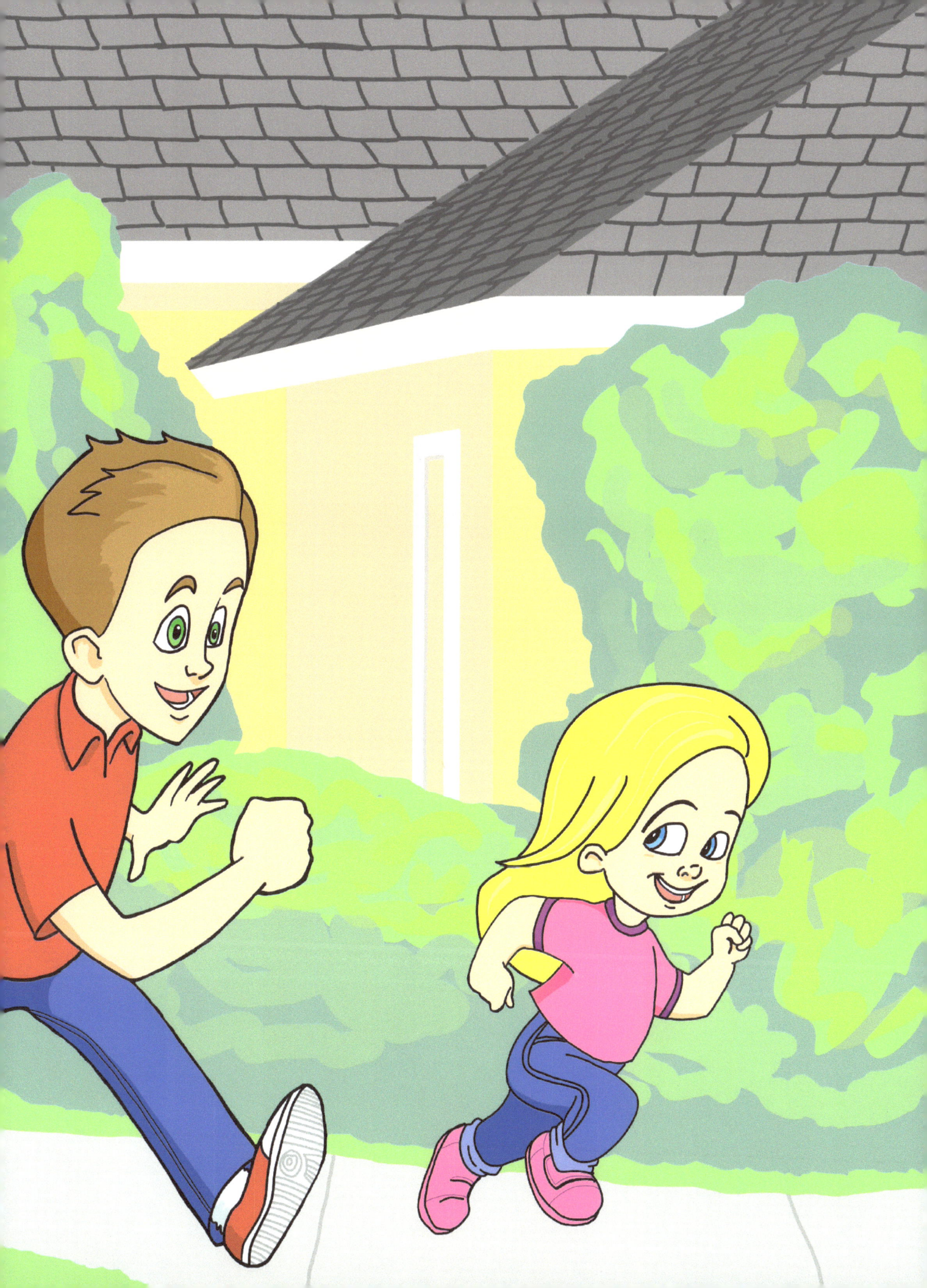

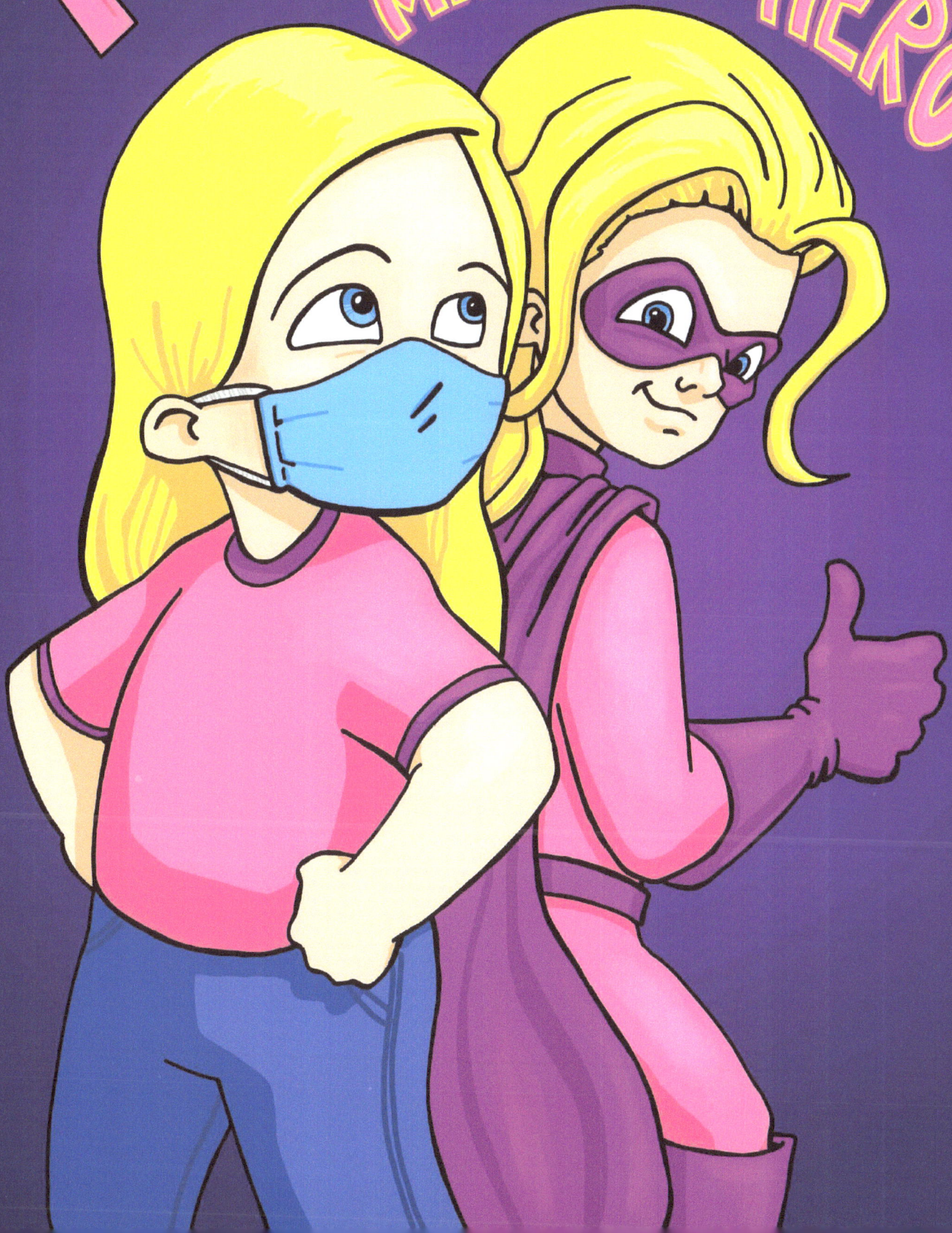

"I wish I had superpowers," Juliette thought.
There are dragons to slay. There are fights to be fought."

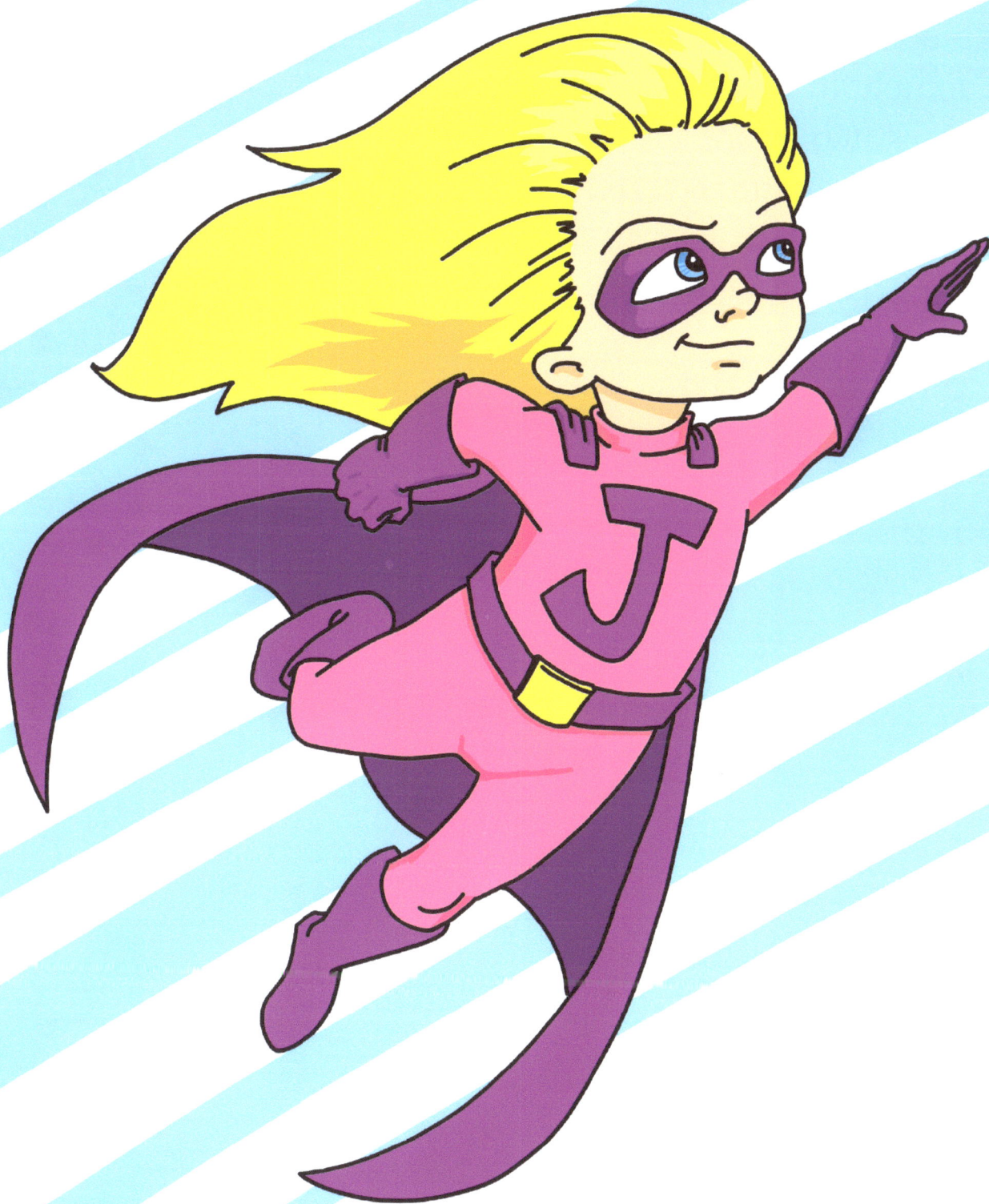

"With my cape on my back and a mask on my face,
I can go and do good things all over the place."

When her mother walked in with some cloth and elastic,
Juliette guessed it was something fantastic.

"What are you making?
Is it blue? Is it green?
Is it somebody's costume for next Halloween?
Are you stitching some socks?
Are we having some guests?
Are they gifts or stuffed monkeys,
some shorts or a dress?"

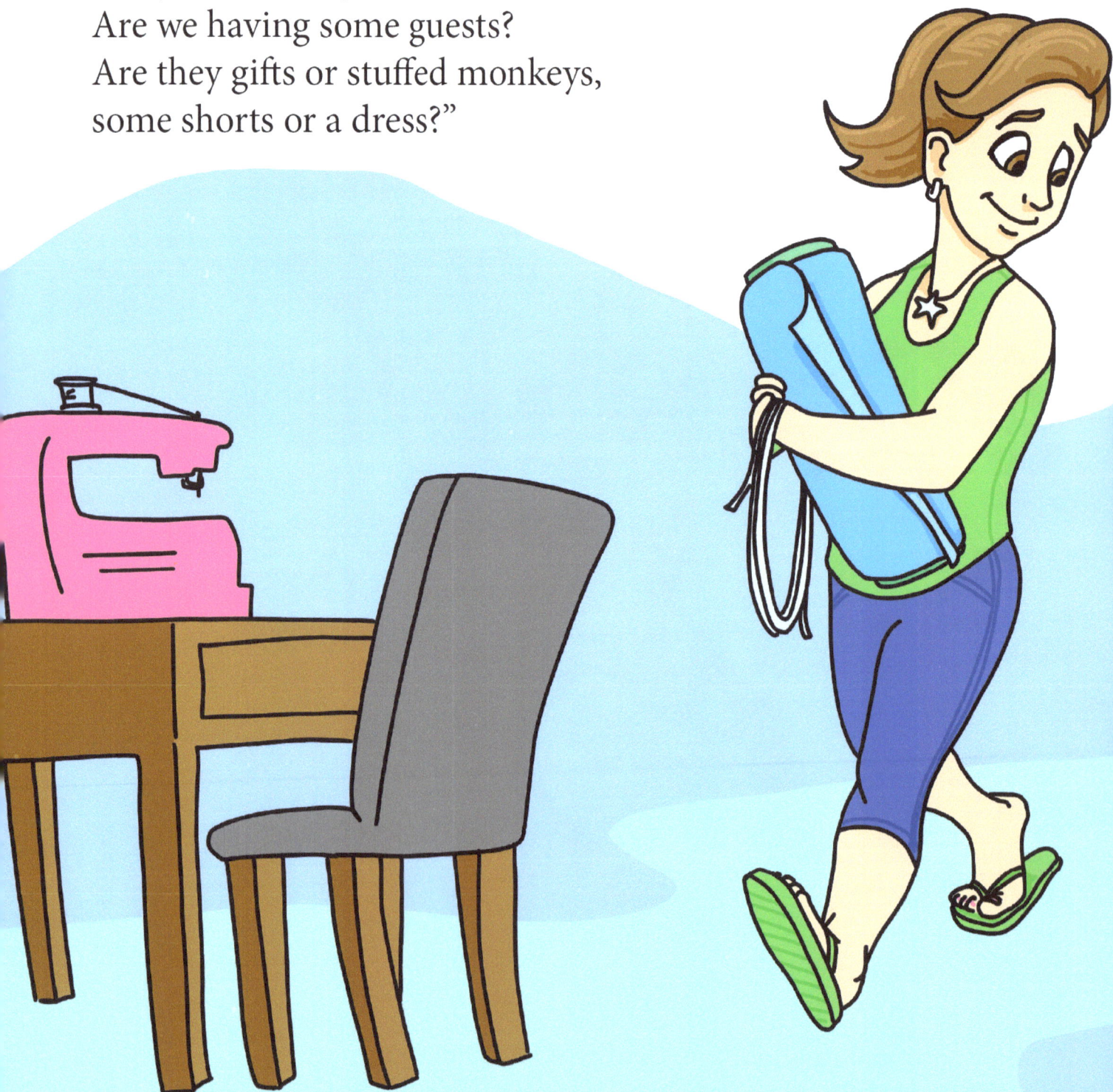

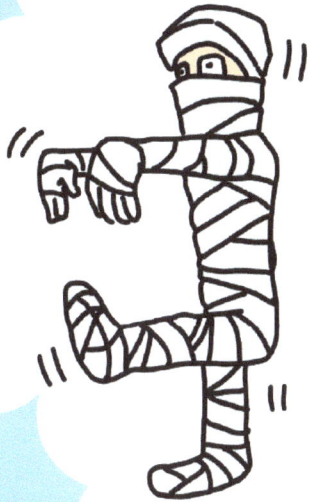

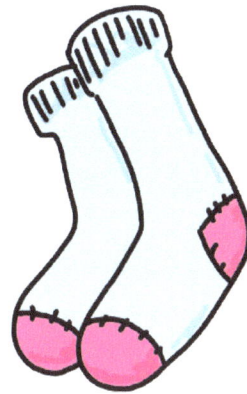

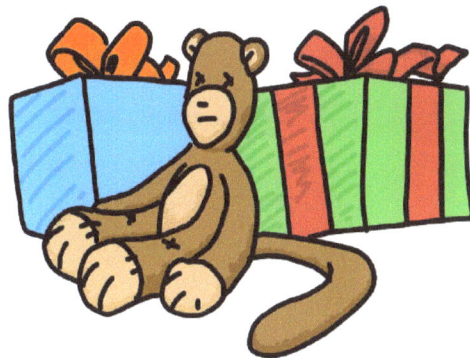

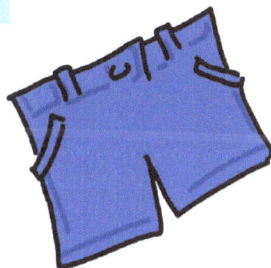

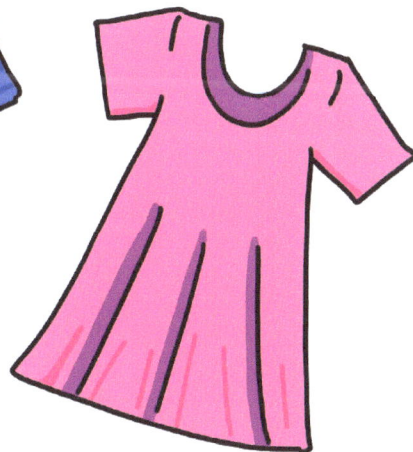

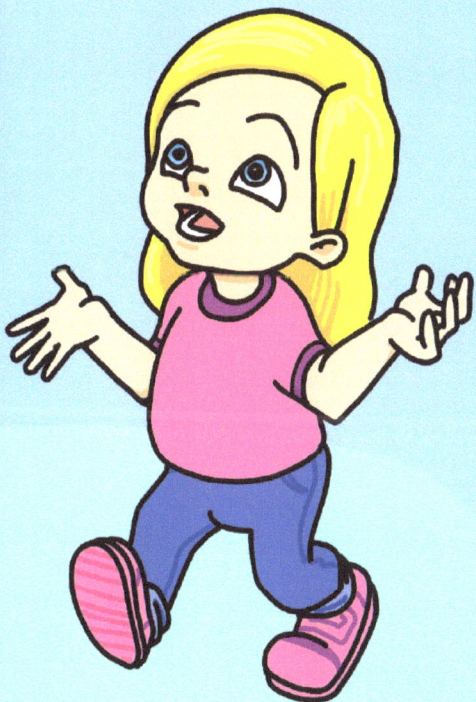

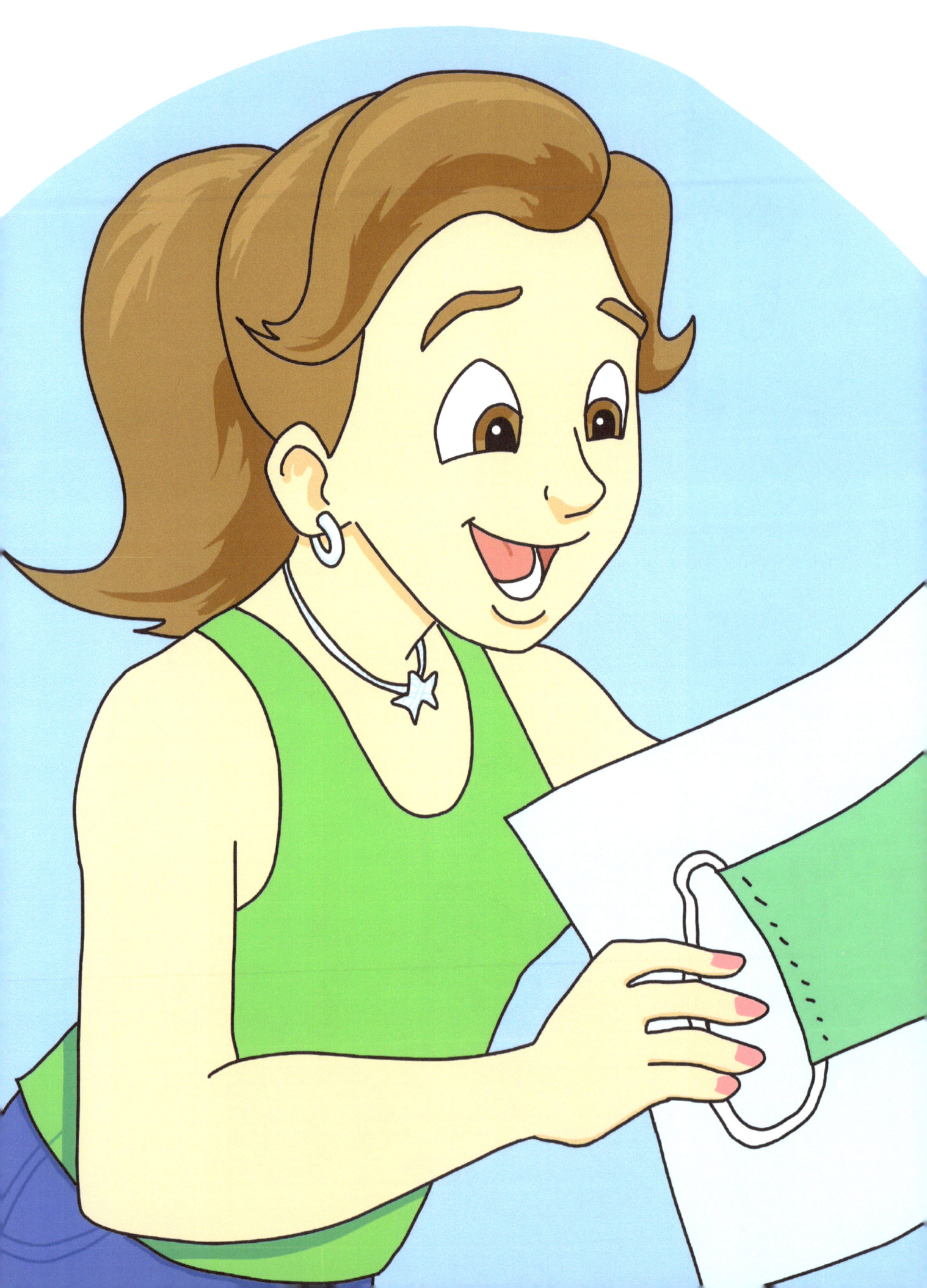

Juliette's mother winked an eye with a smile.
"It's a fun little project. It's something worthwhile.
I'm making an outfit that all heroes wear.
It helps to protect you and shows that you care."

She held up a pattern. It had four right angles.
It looked very plain. A simple rectangle.

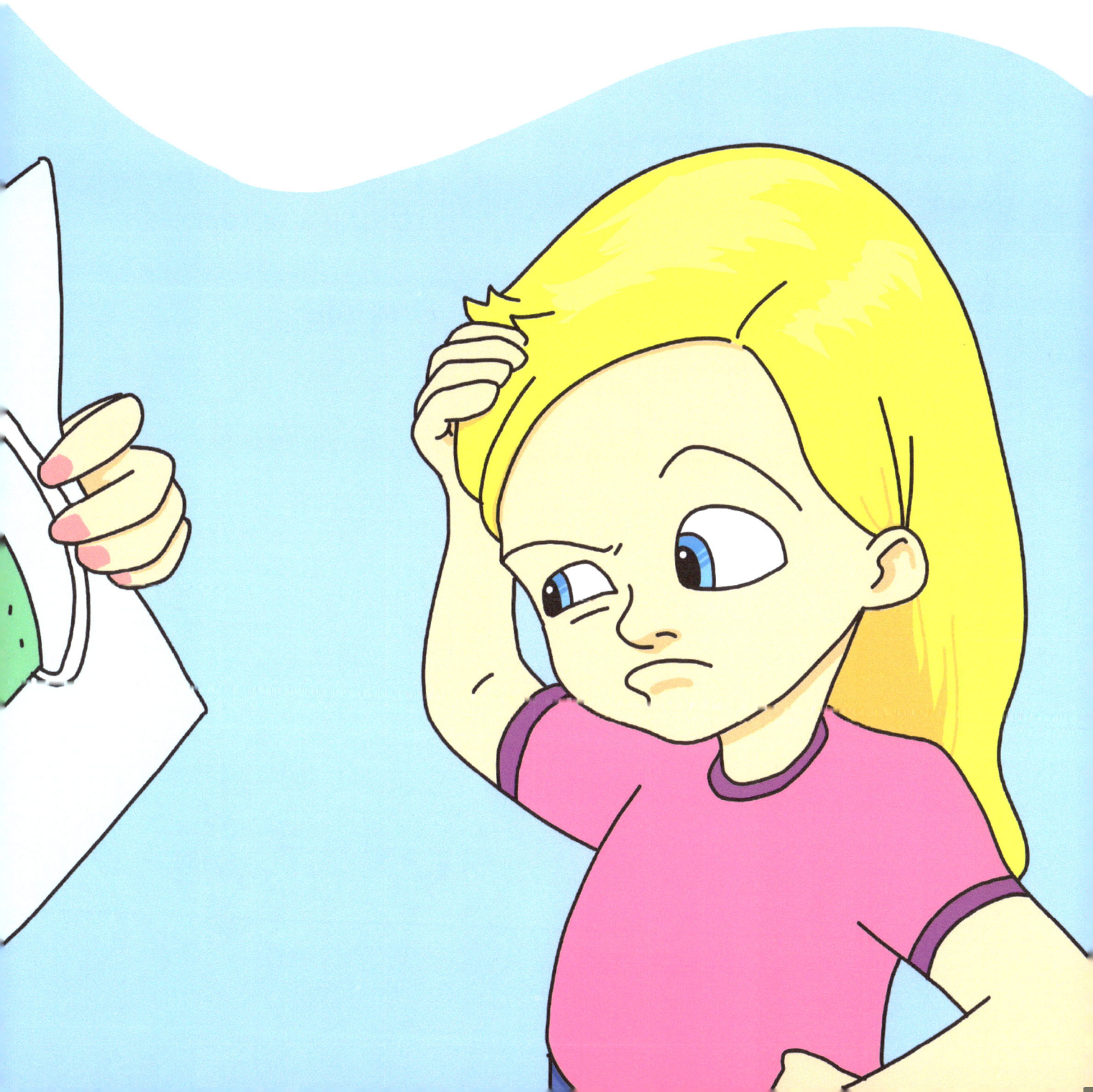

Two pieces of fabric
lay one on another.
"Now watch what I do,"
said Juliette's mother.

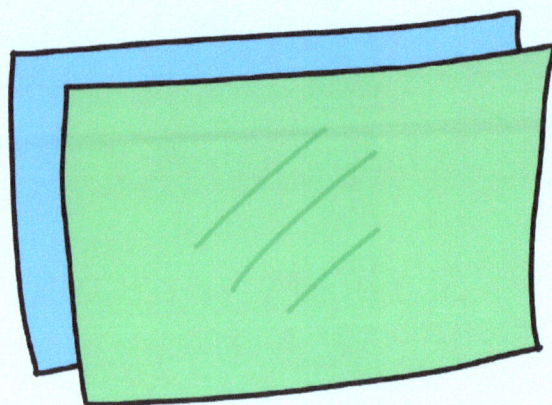

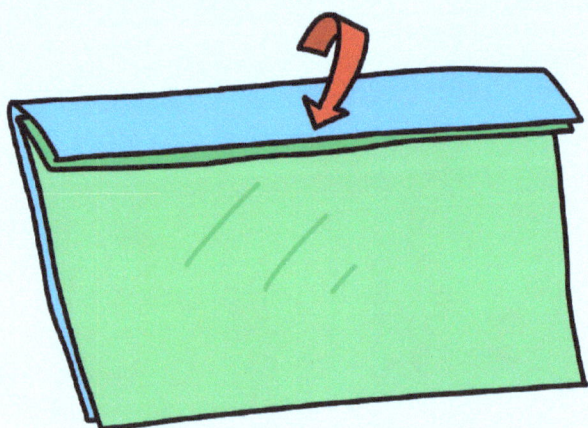

"I fold in the edges,
creating a border.

First top...

and then bottom,

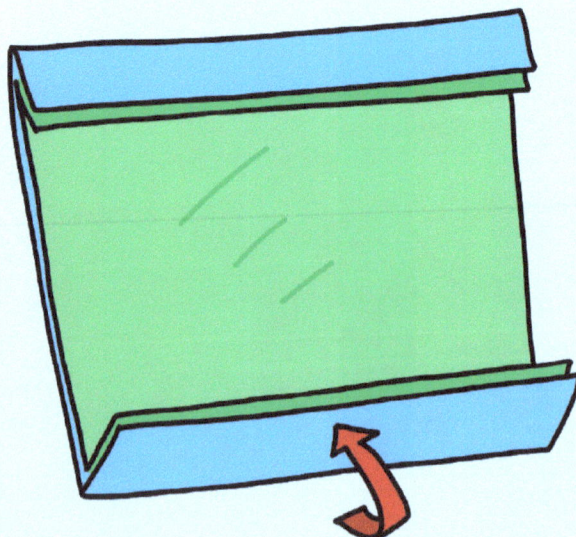

then the sides in that order."

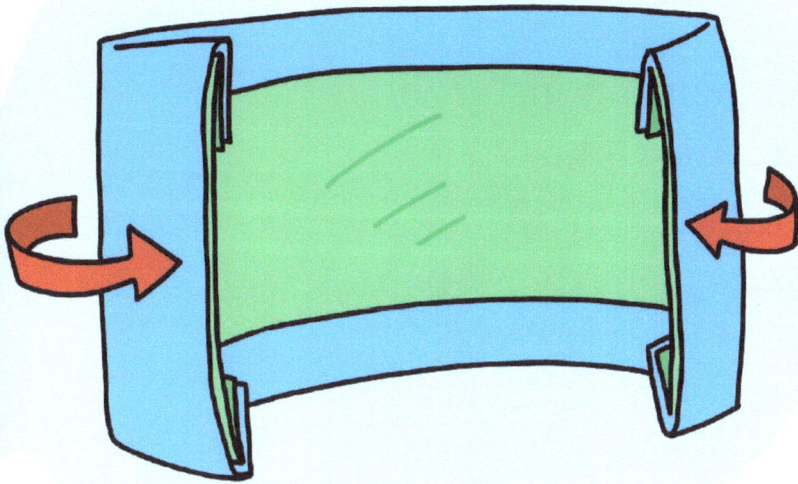

"Then we sew and we stitch, leaving just enough space,
to thread some elastic and tie it in place."

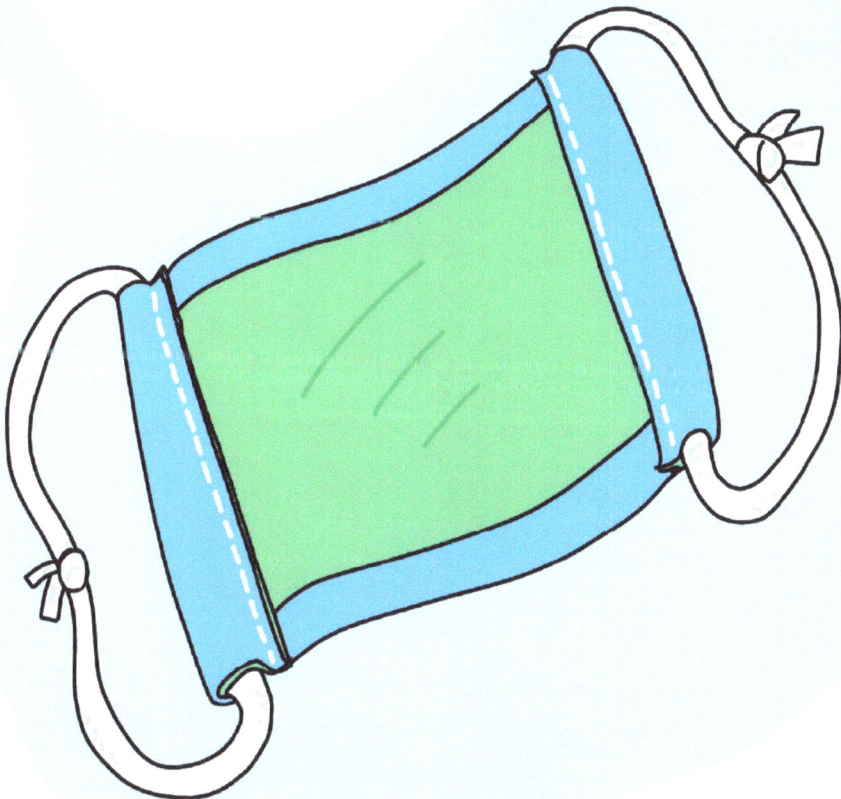

"What is this creation?"
young Juliette asked.
Her mom held it up...

"It's a Superhero's mask!"

She adjusted the strings so the mask fit just right.
It covered Jules' smile. It wasn't too tight.
Juliette wondered, "Why do we wear them?
Do we each have our own? Is it OK to share them?"

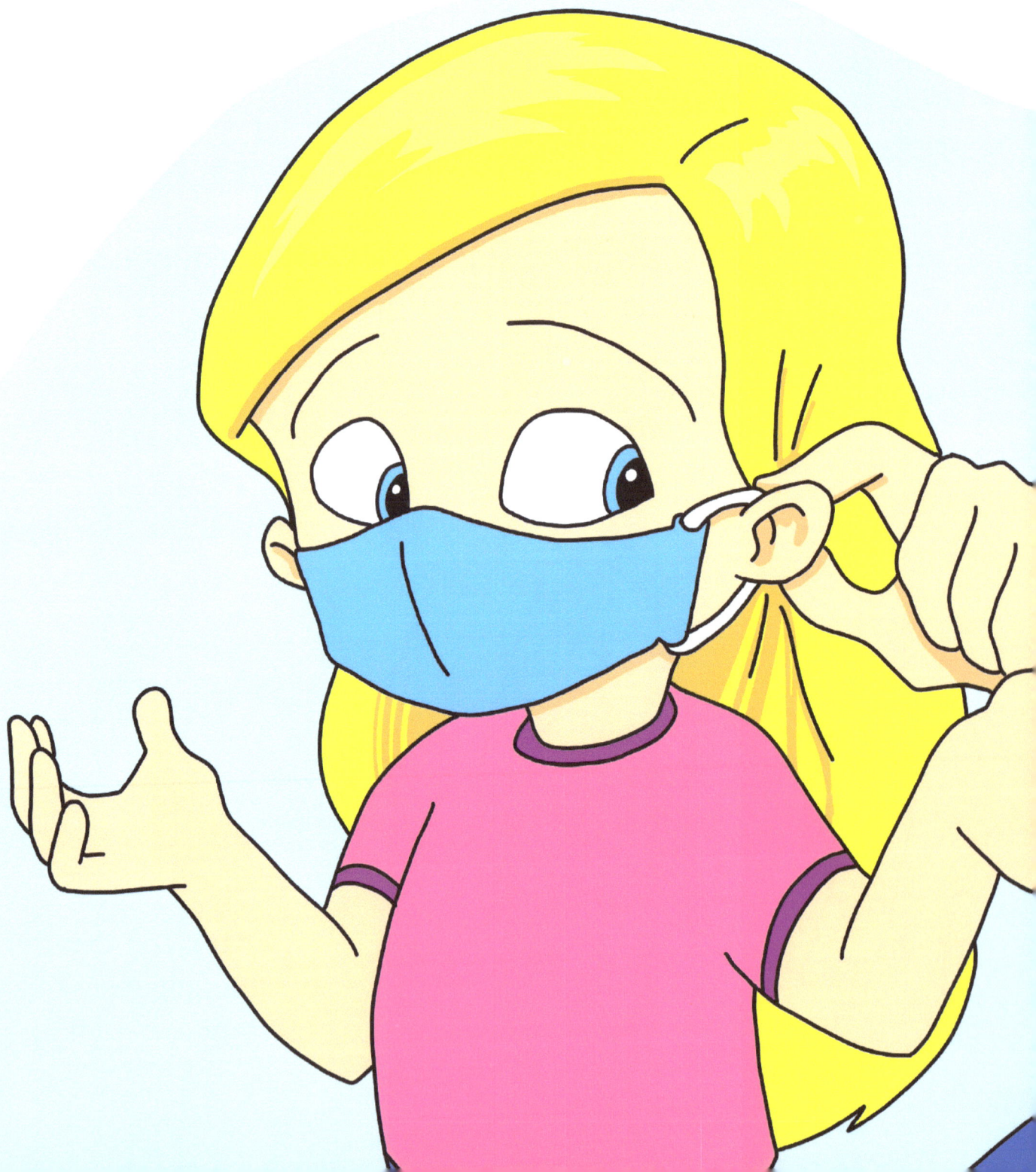

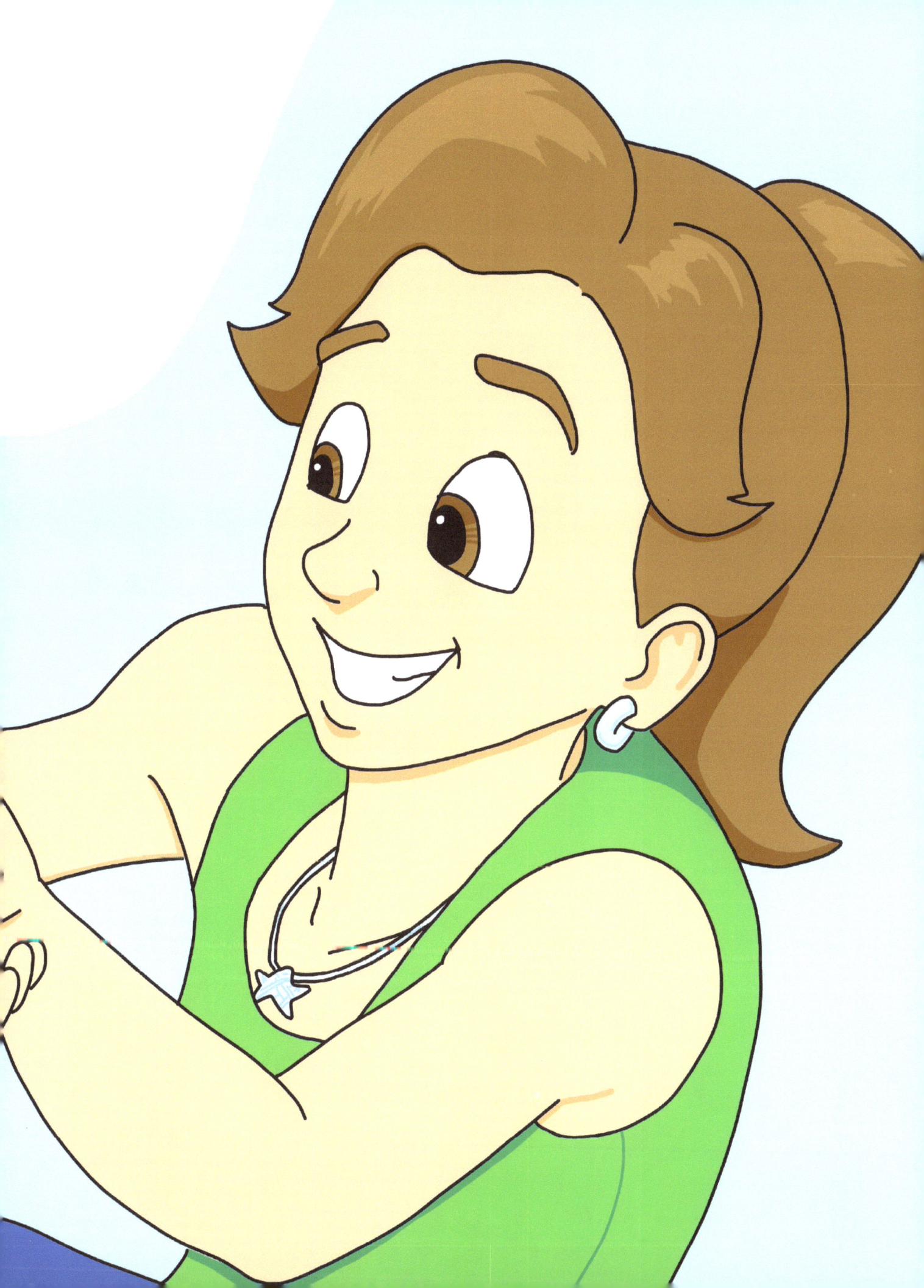

"Masks are a shield," said Juliette's mother.
"Carried by knights, and by kids like your brother."

"Some germs that surround us
can make people sick.
They sneak in when you breathe.
It can happen quite quick."

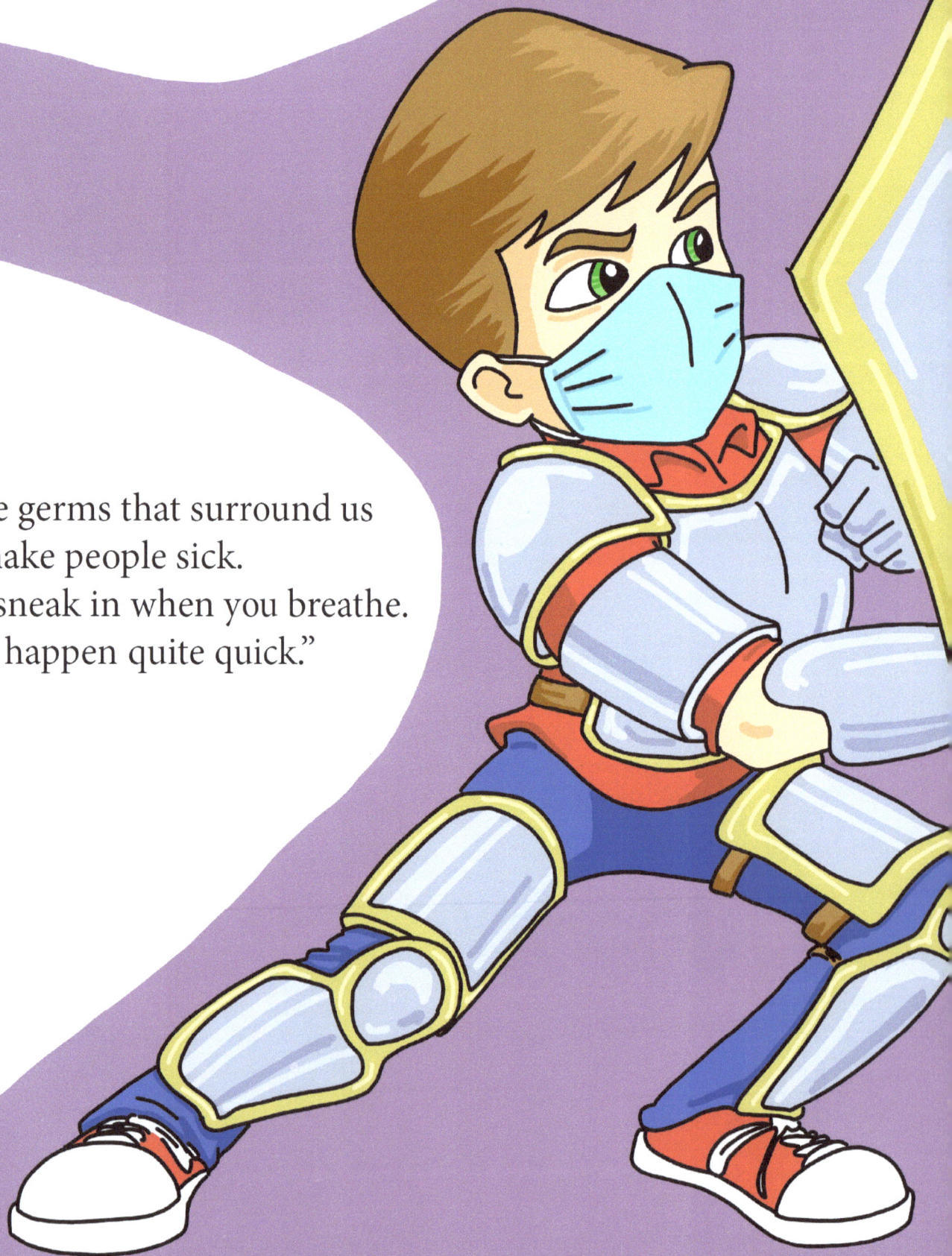

GERMS

"Wearing a mask gives you added protection.
It's stops every bug, from every direction."

"And if you feel germy a mask can help, too!
It shields your friends. They won't catch germs from you."

Juliette's eyes reflected her smile.
"I like my new mask. I like my new style.
I could join the police, be a dancer, a doctor,
a dentist, a parent, a teacher, a shopper."

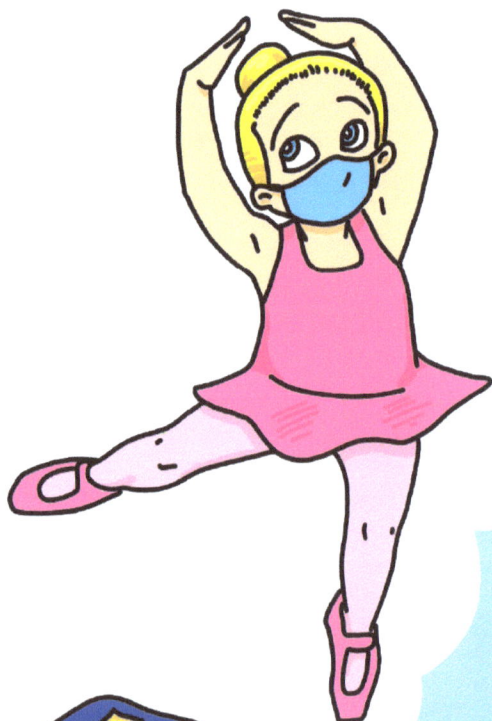

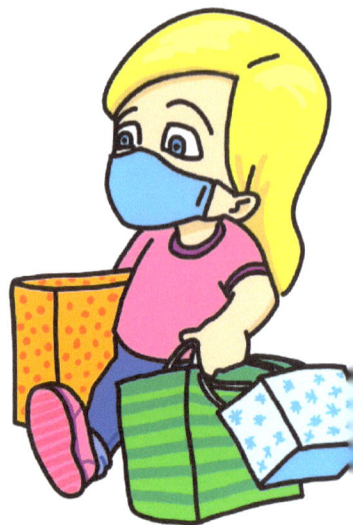

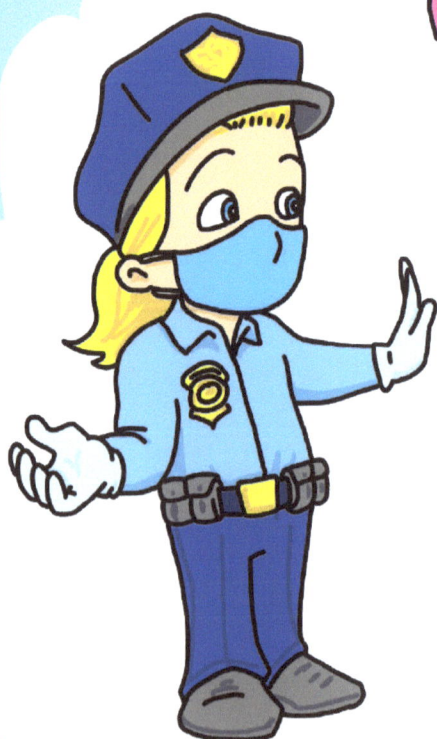

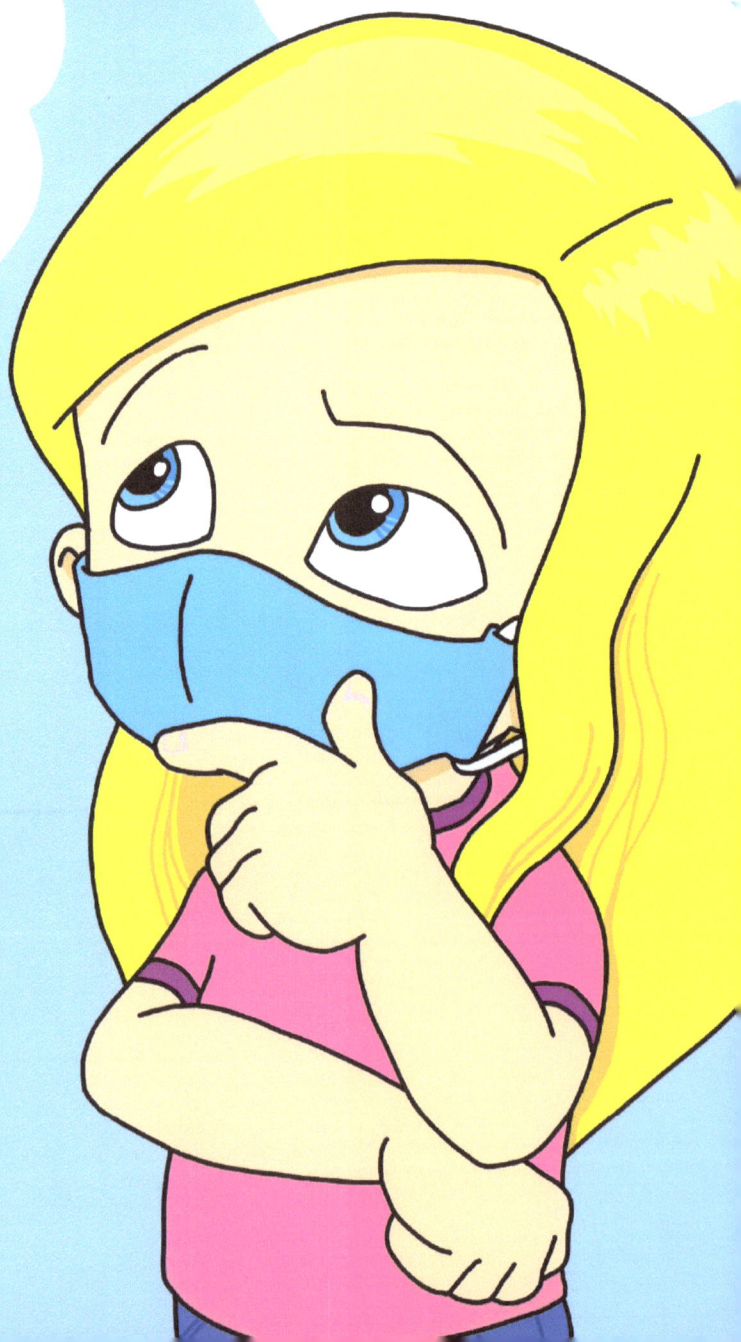

"With my new mask, I can shout, I can sing,
I can study the stars, I can do anything!"

What else can you teach me?
What more should I do
to keep myself healthy
and help others, too?"

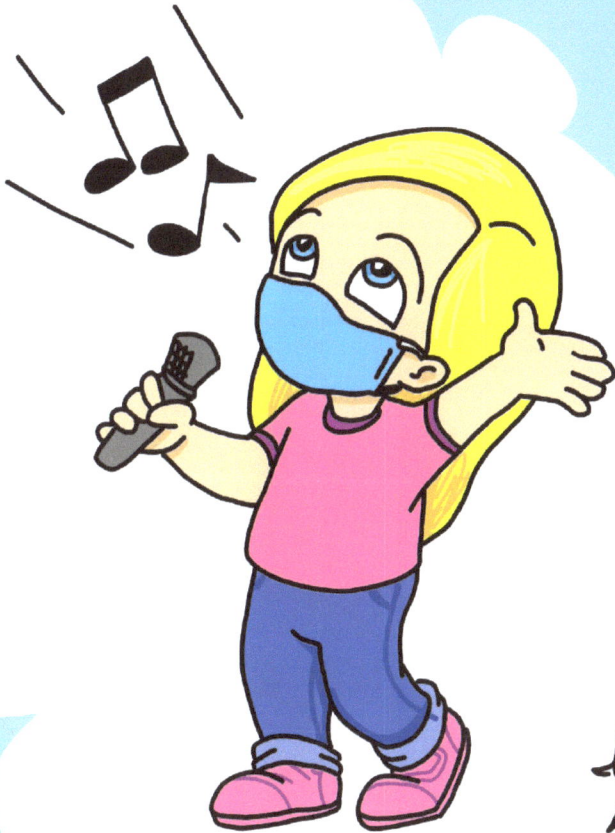

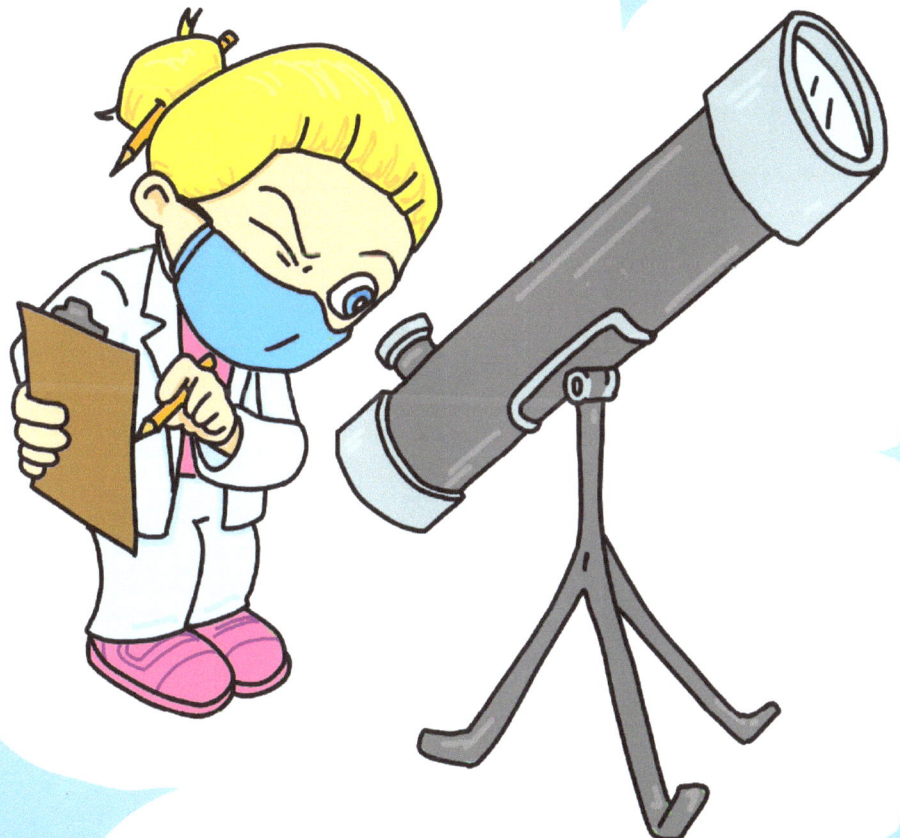

Juliette's mother loved her persistence.
"I have one more tip: Be aware of your distance."

"I know you love hugging, but during bug season, don't get too close. And here is the reason."

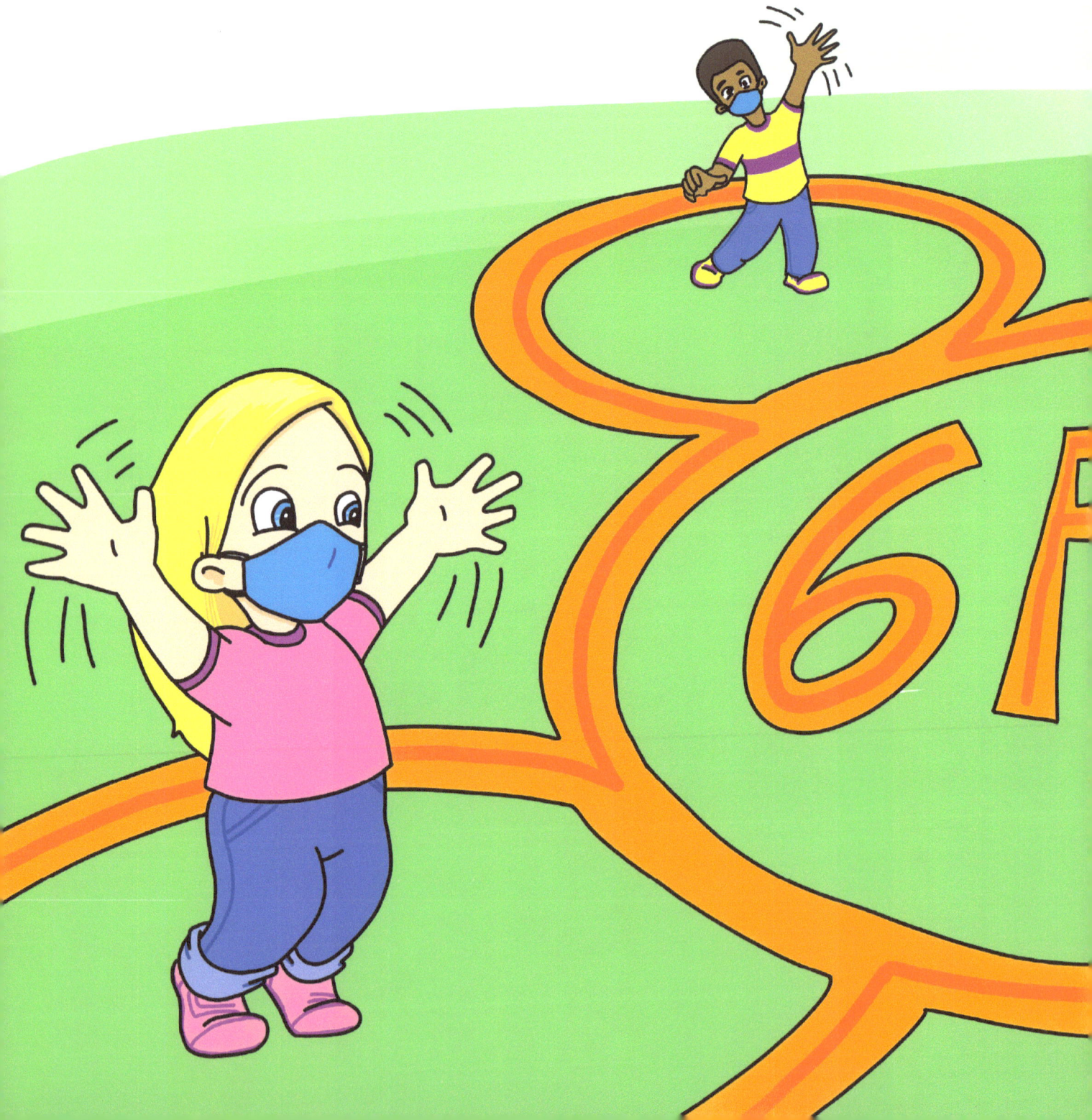

"The germs in our bodies can float through the air.
They can land on your nose. They can dance on your hair."

"Stand a bit further away from your friend.
The bugs will get tired. Their travels will end."

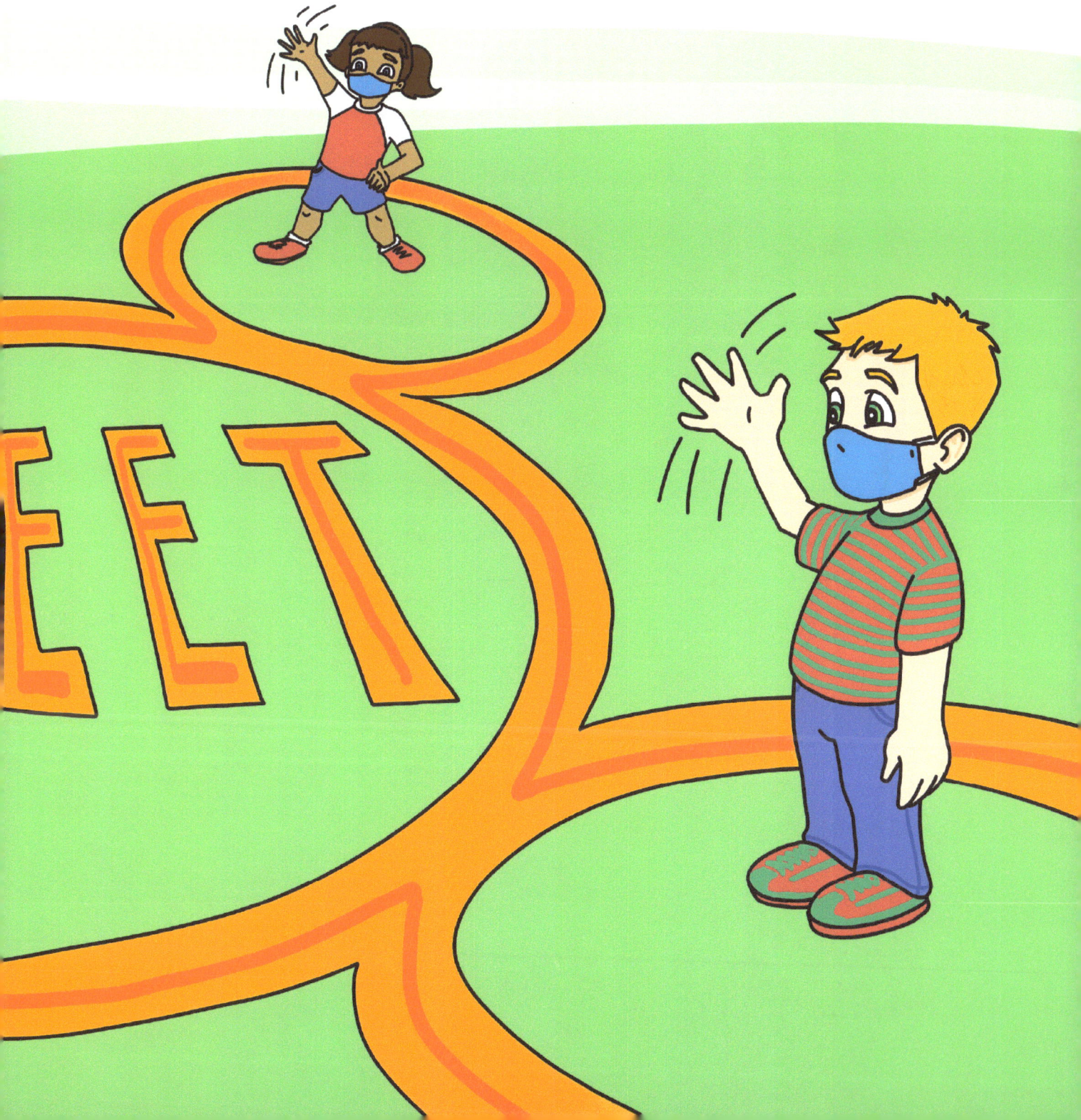

Juliette laughed as she walked toward the door.
"I'm off to find heroes, perhaps to make more!"

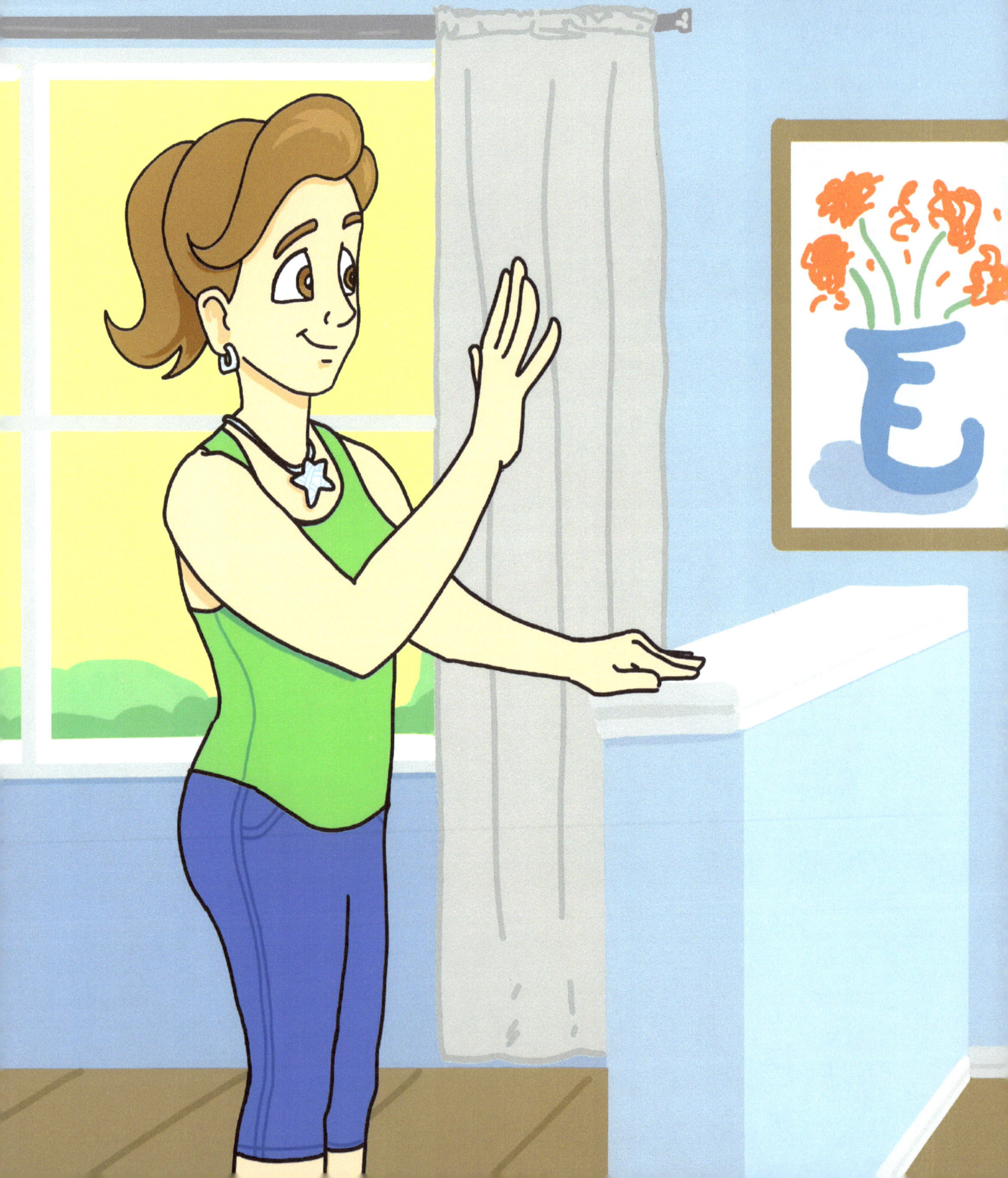

She made a discovery as she skipped down the stair...

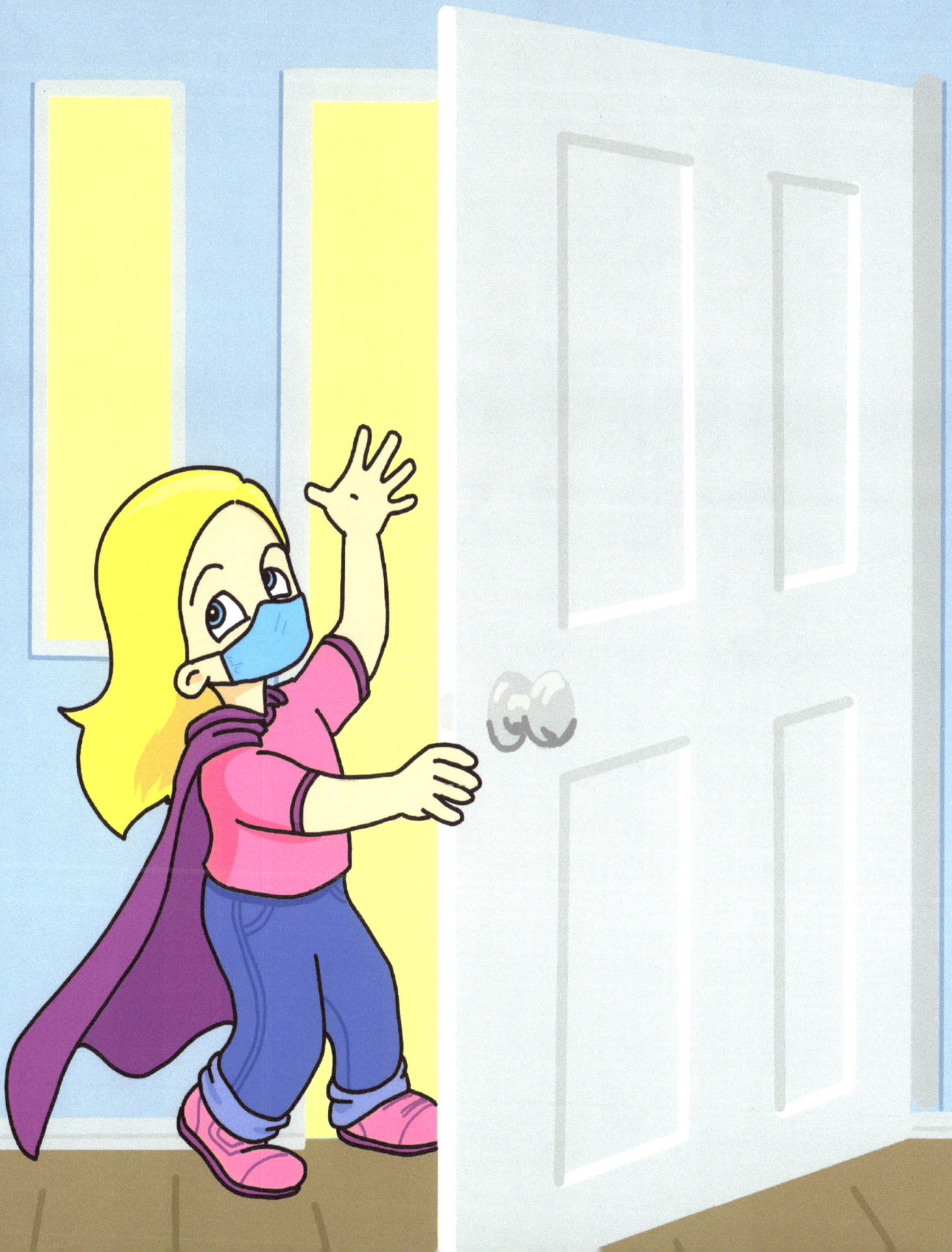

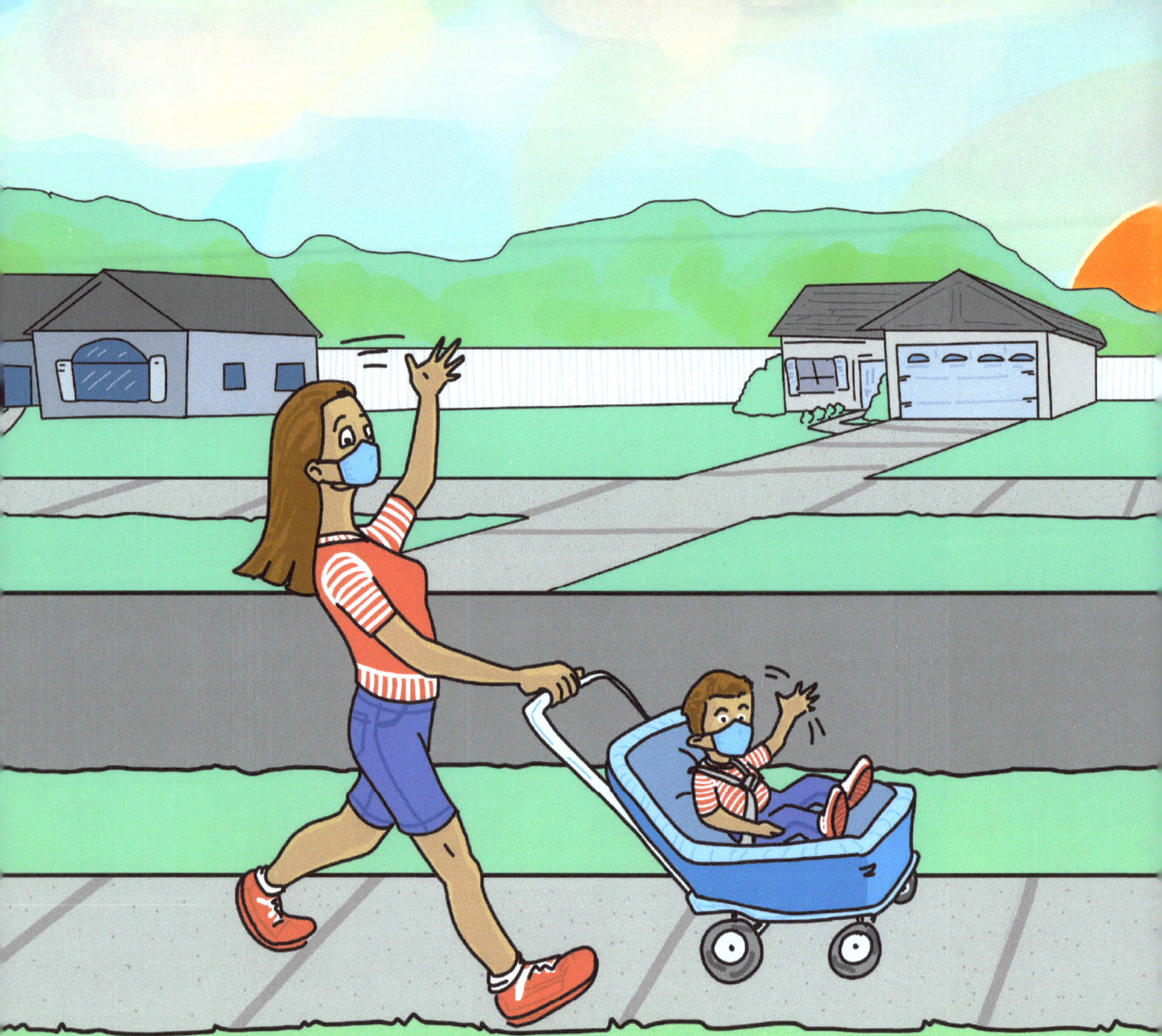

The heroes she sought could be found everywhere.

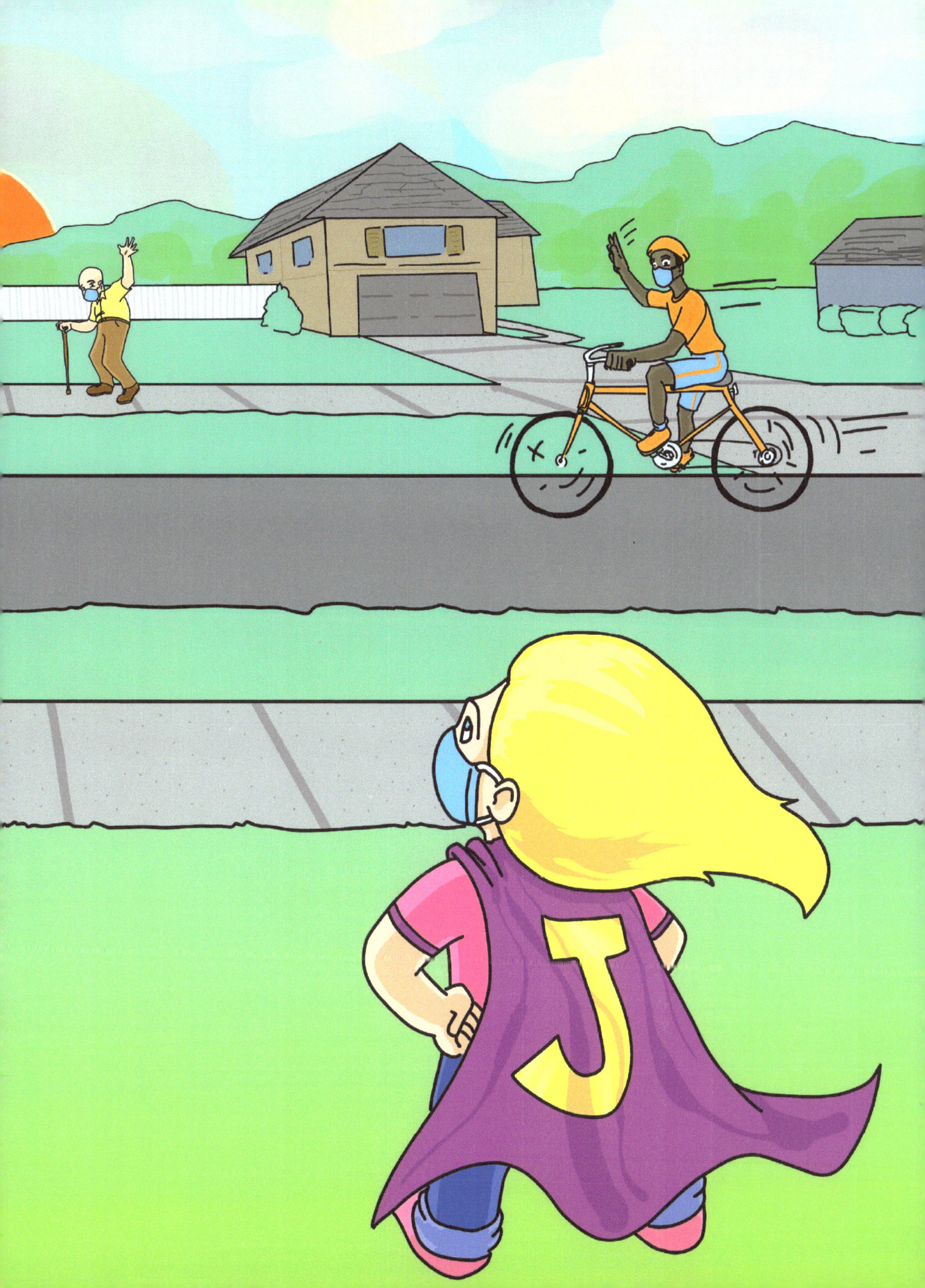

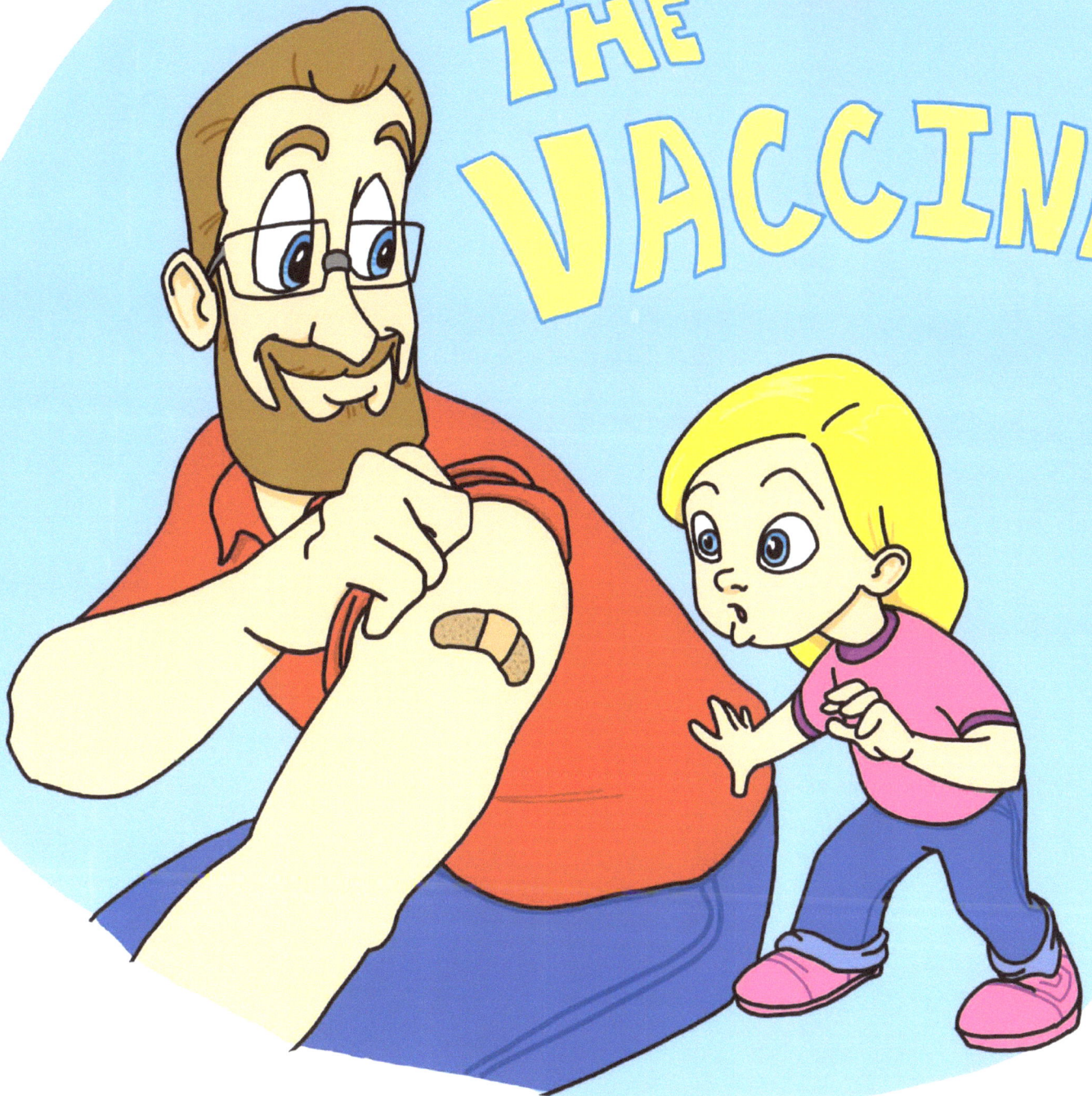

"I'm off to the doctor's," said Juliette's Dad.
To get some protection from bugs that are bad.
We mask, and we distance. We keep our hands clean.
Now all that we need is the latest vaccine."

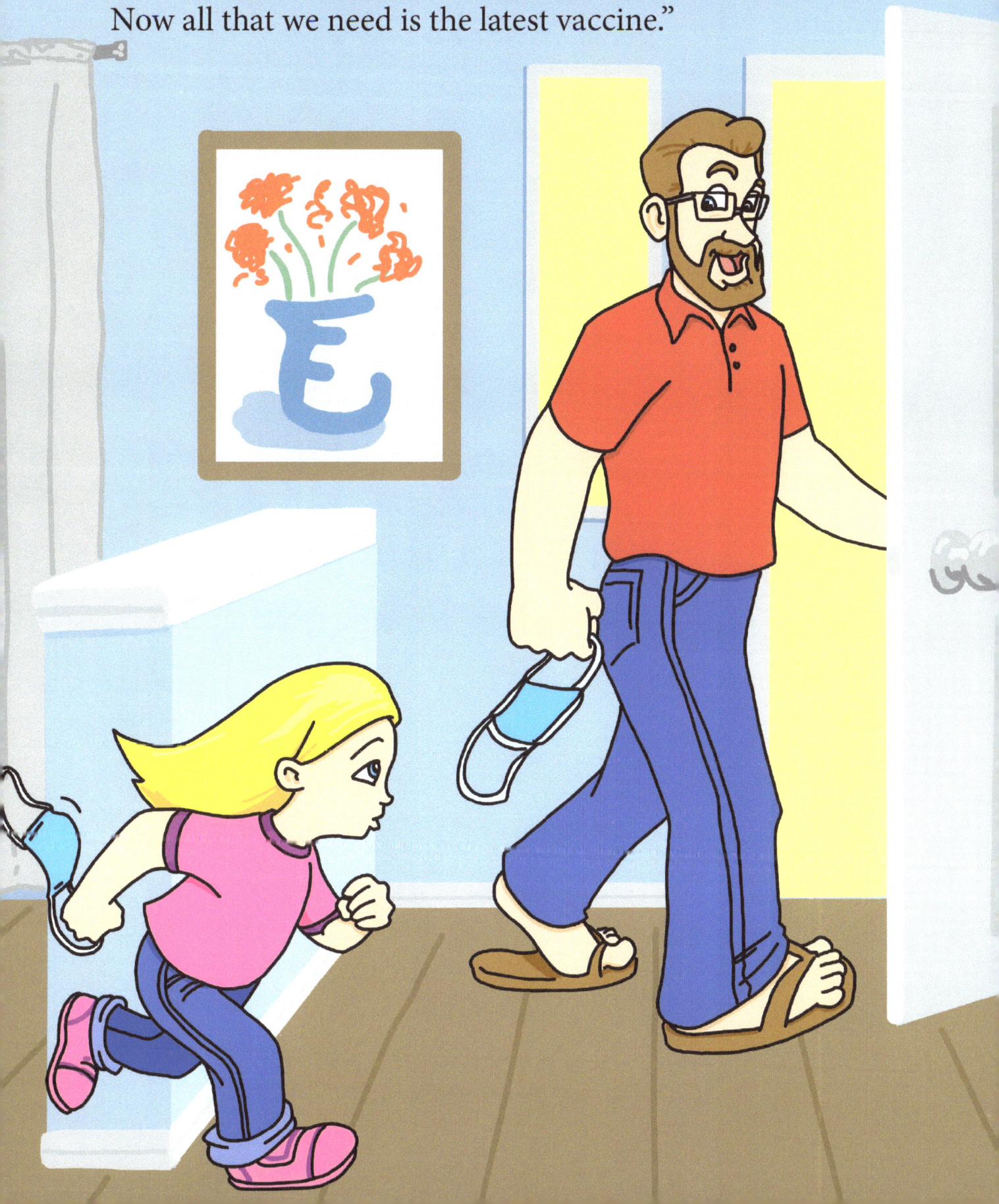

"What's a vaccine?"
young Juliette asked.
"Is it like washing your hands
and wearing a mask?"

"Put simply," he said,
"It's a poke in the arm.
They call it a 'shot.'
It will protect you from harm."

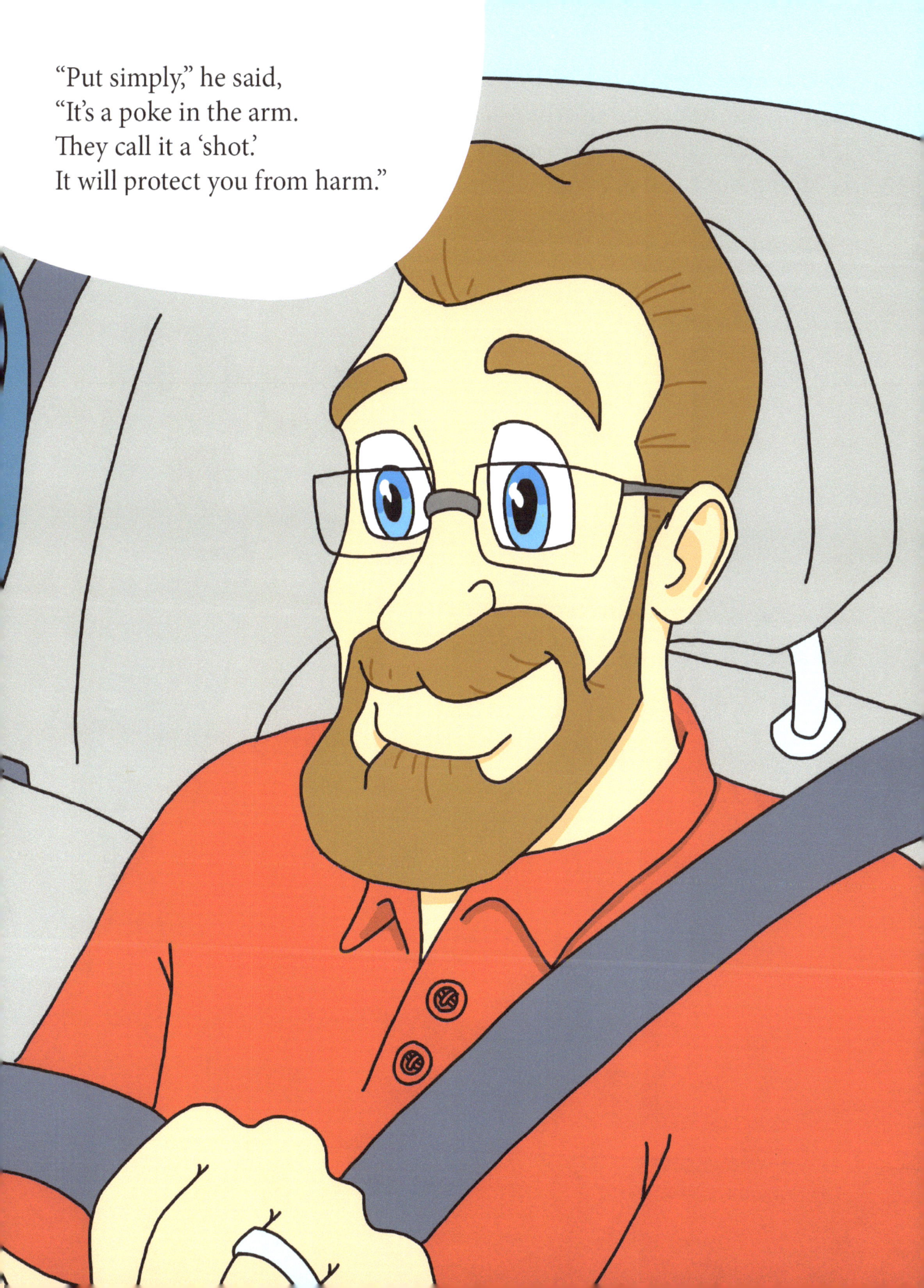

"Our bodies have soldiers," Dad went on to explain.
"They work to defend us from sickness and pain.
The vaccine tells soldiers to stand and to fight.
To stamp out the bad bugs and make us feel right."

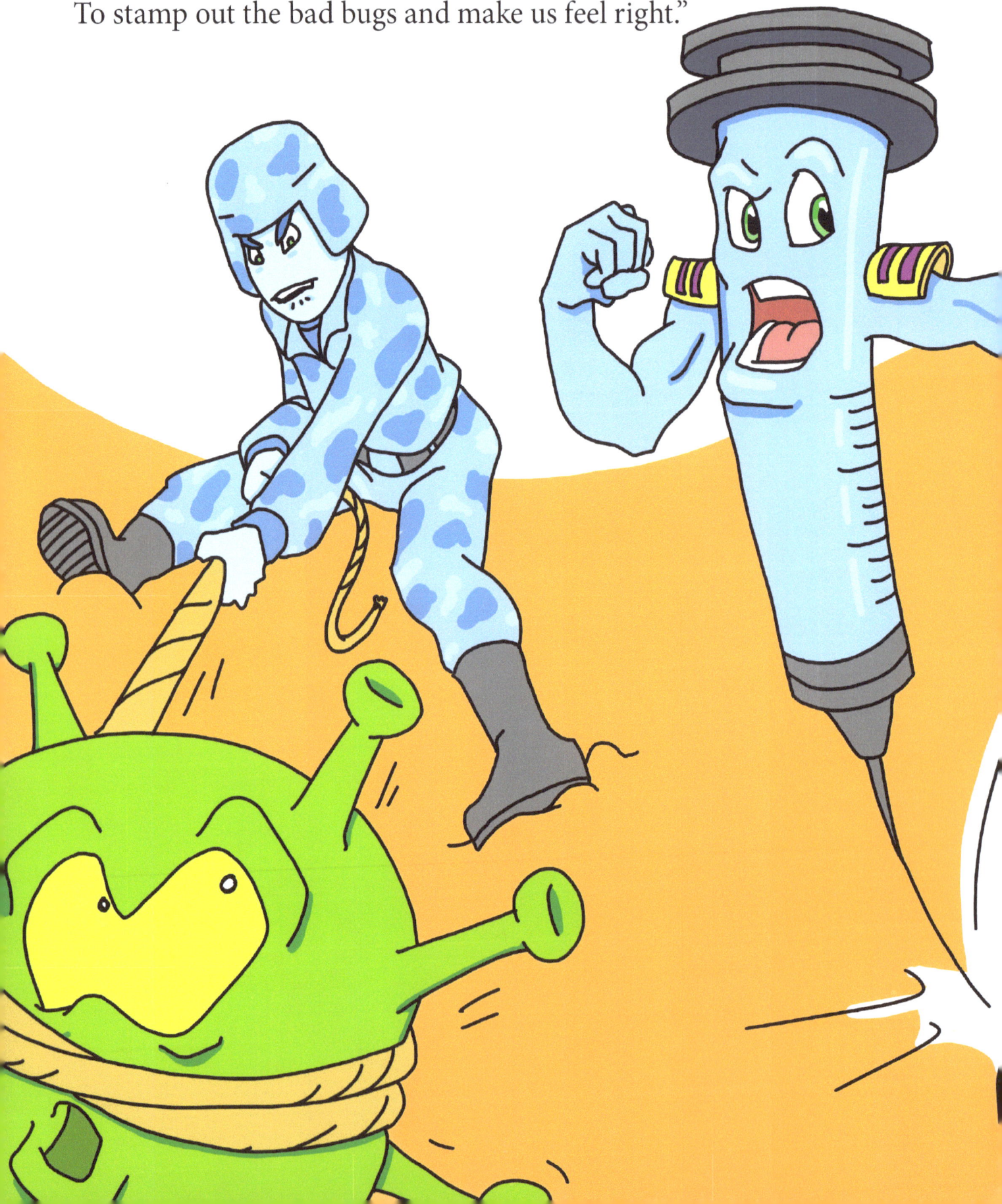

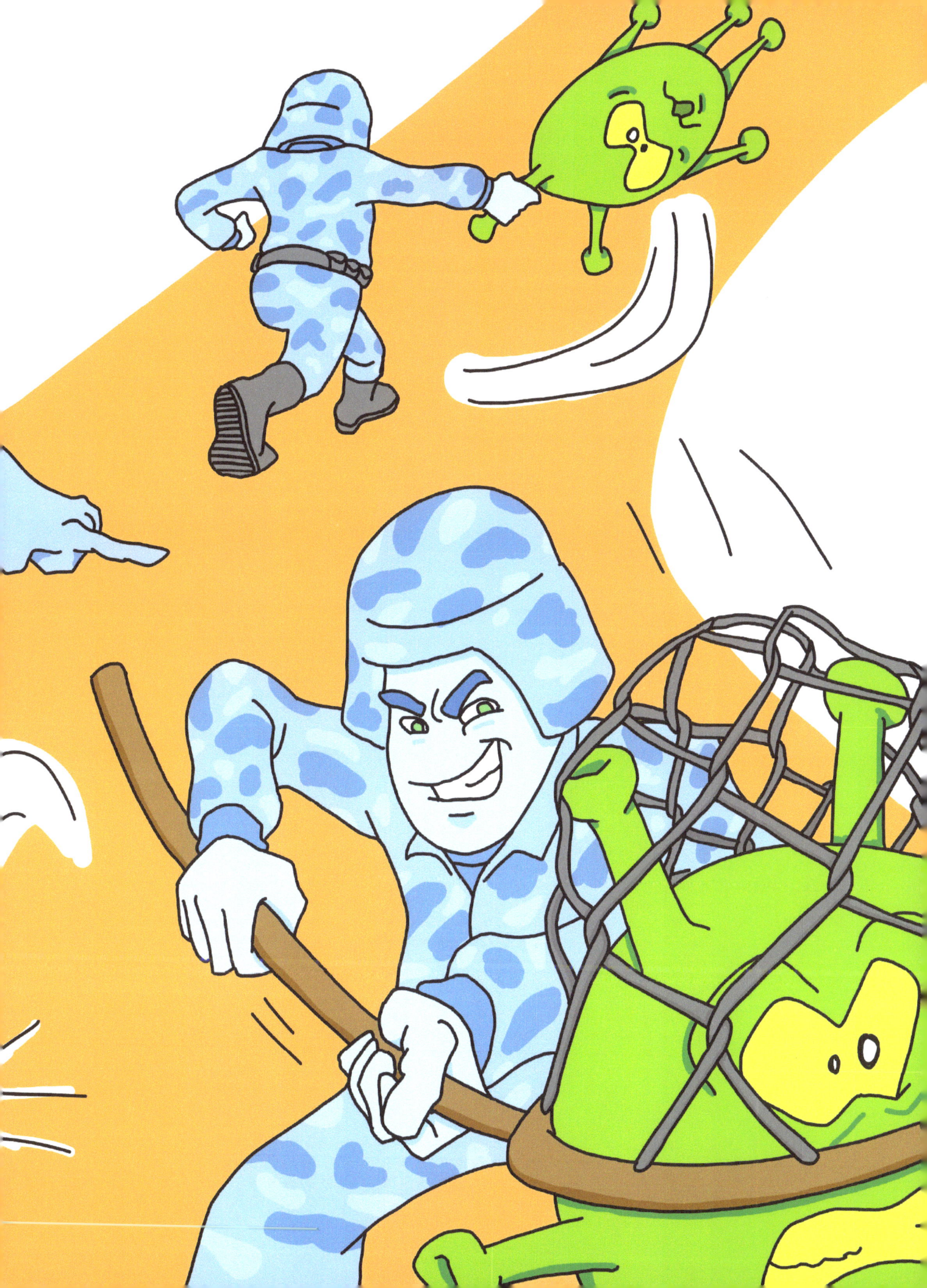

The doctor showed Juliette a tiny glass vial.
After the shot she said, "Rest for a while."

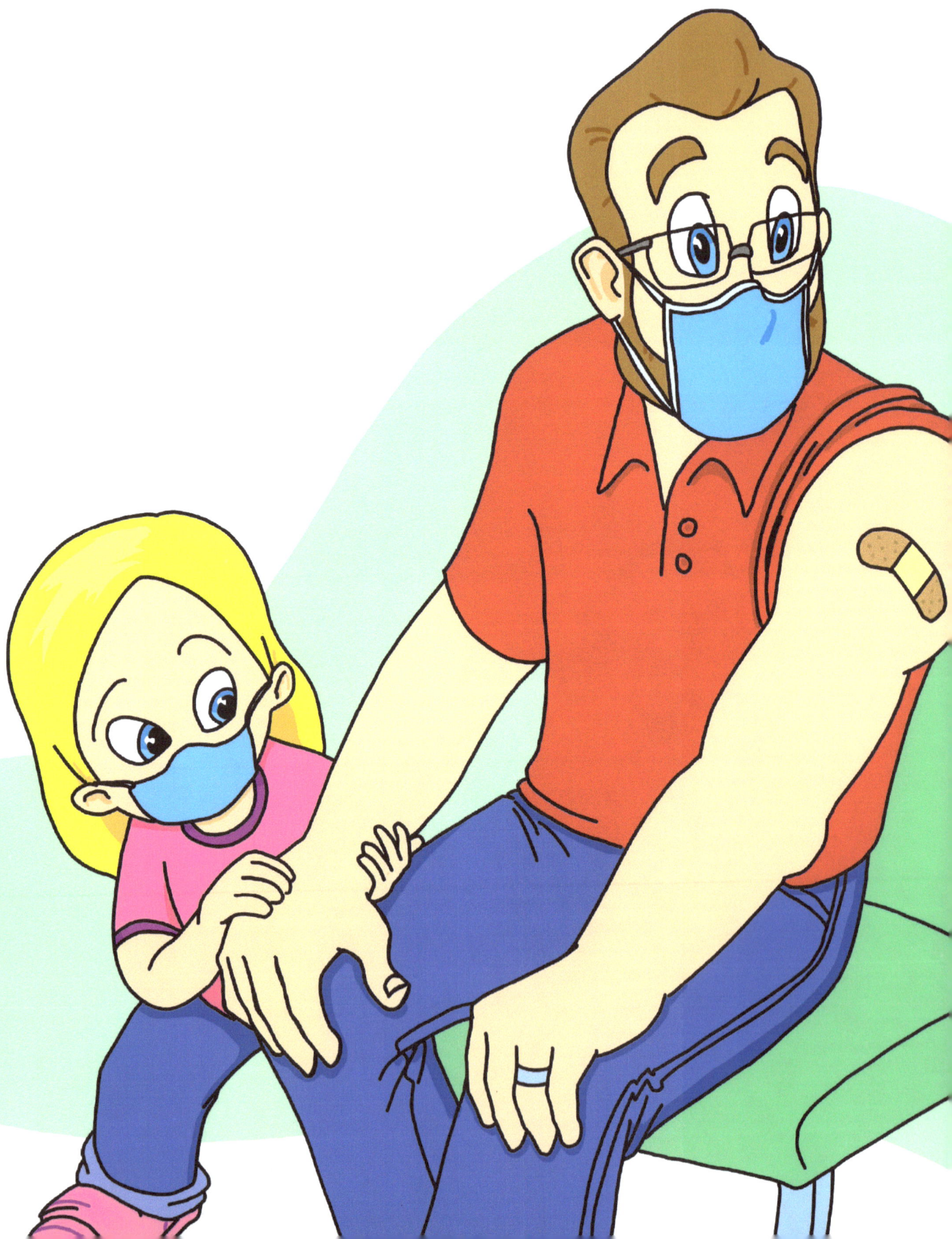

"Dad may feel a bit sore, like a bug might be lurking,
But his soldiers are fighting. The vaccine is working."

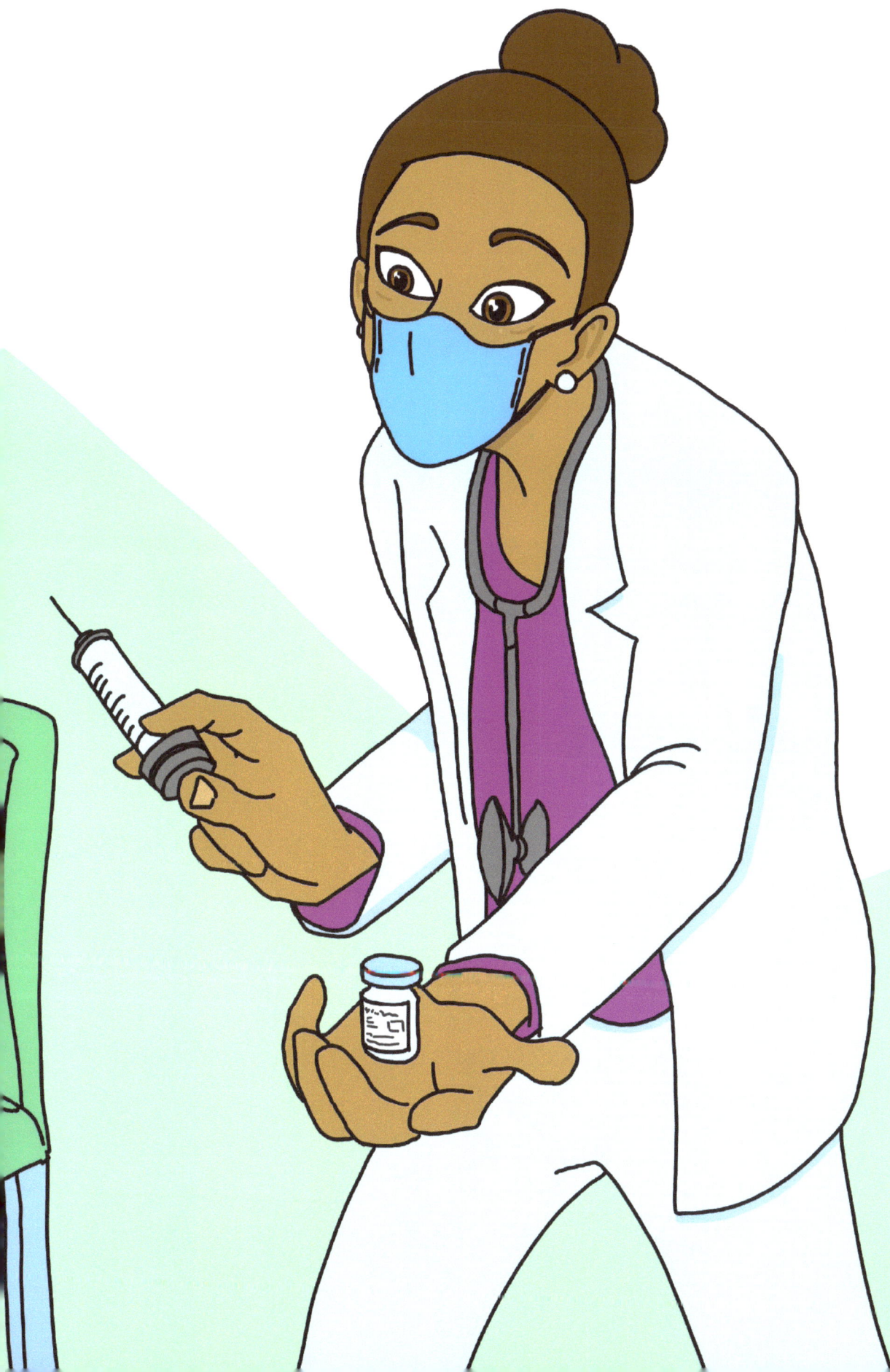

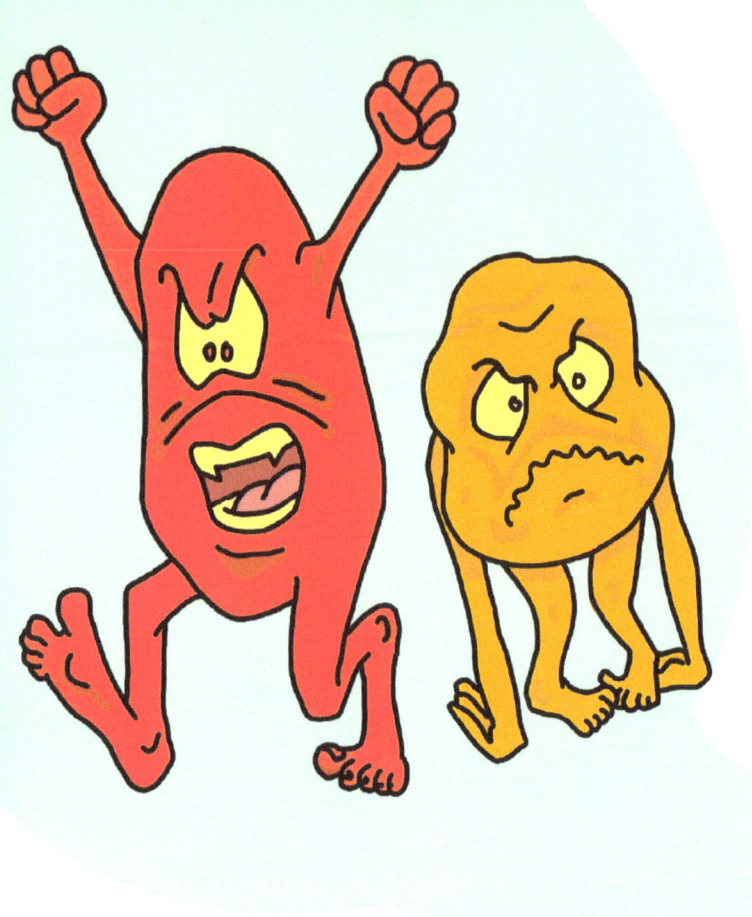

And that's how it happens when new bugs convene.

Scientists study and work to create a vaccine.

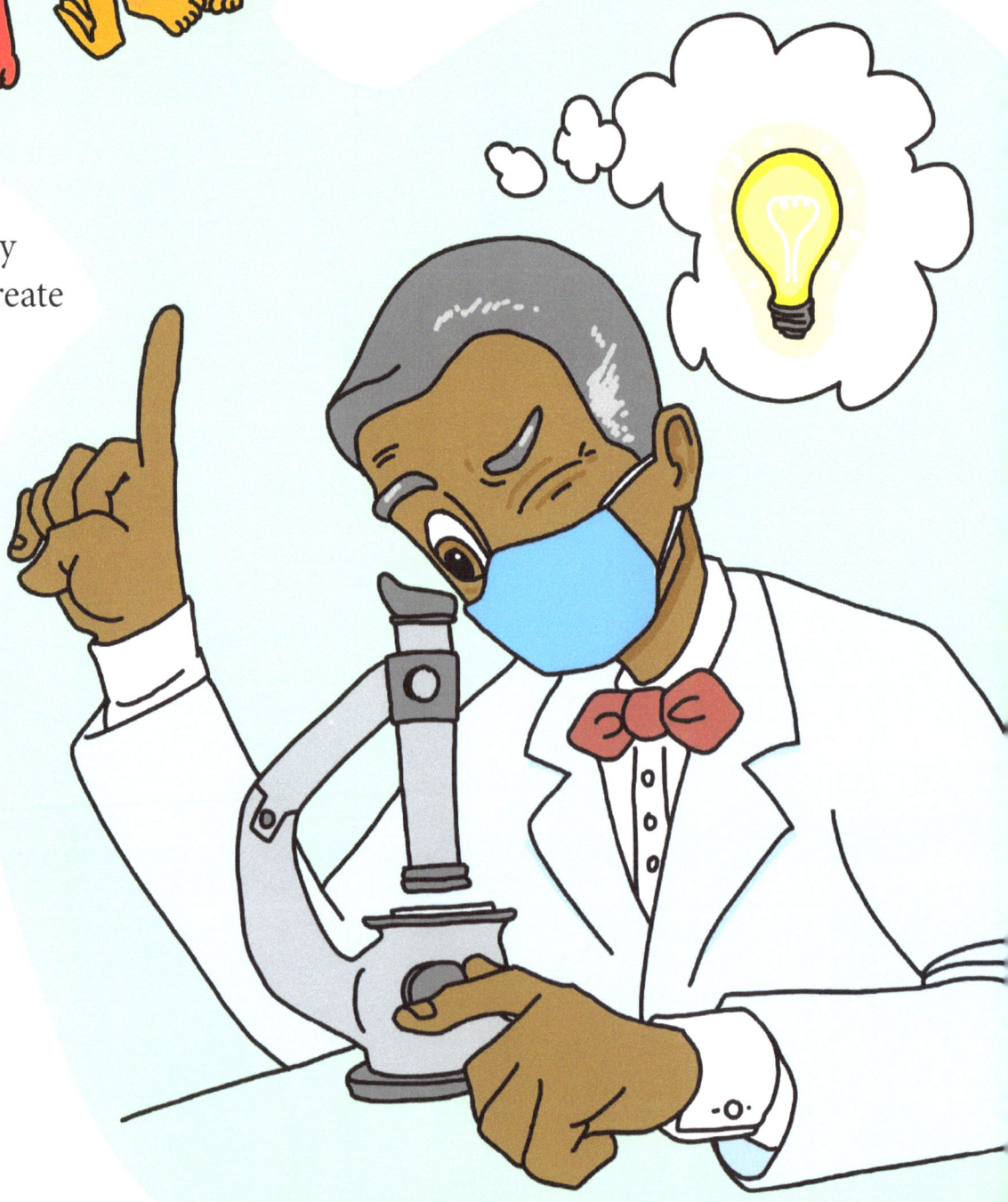

It's carefully tested
and when it is cleared,
we all get the shot...

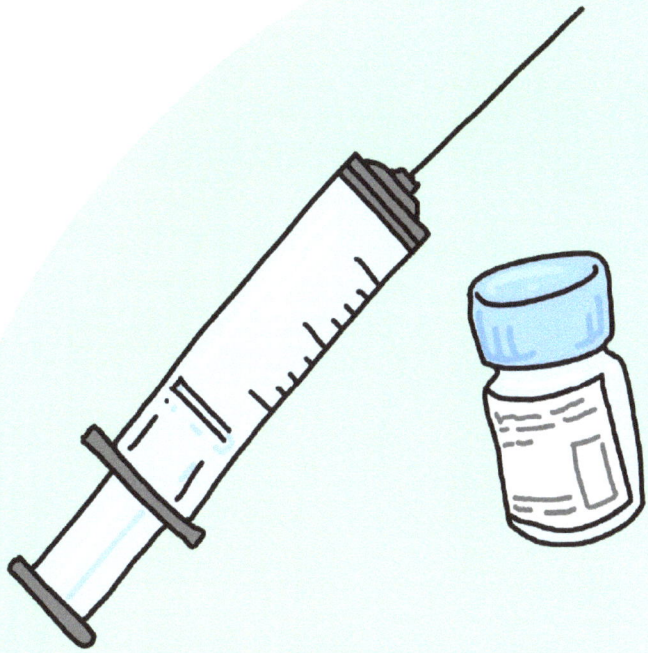

and the bugs disappear!

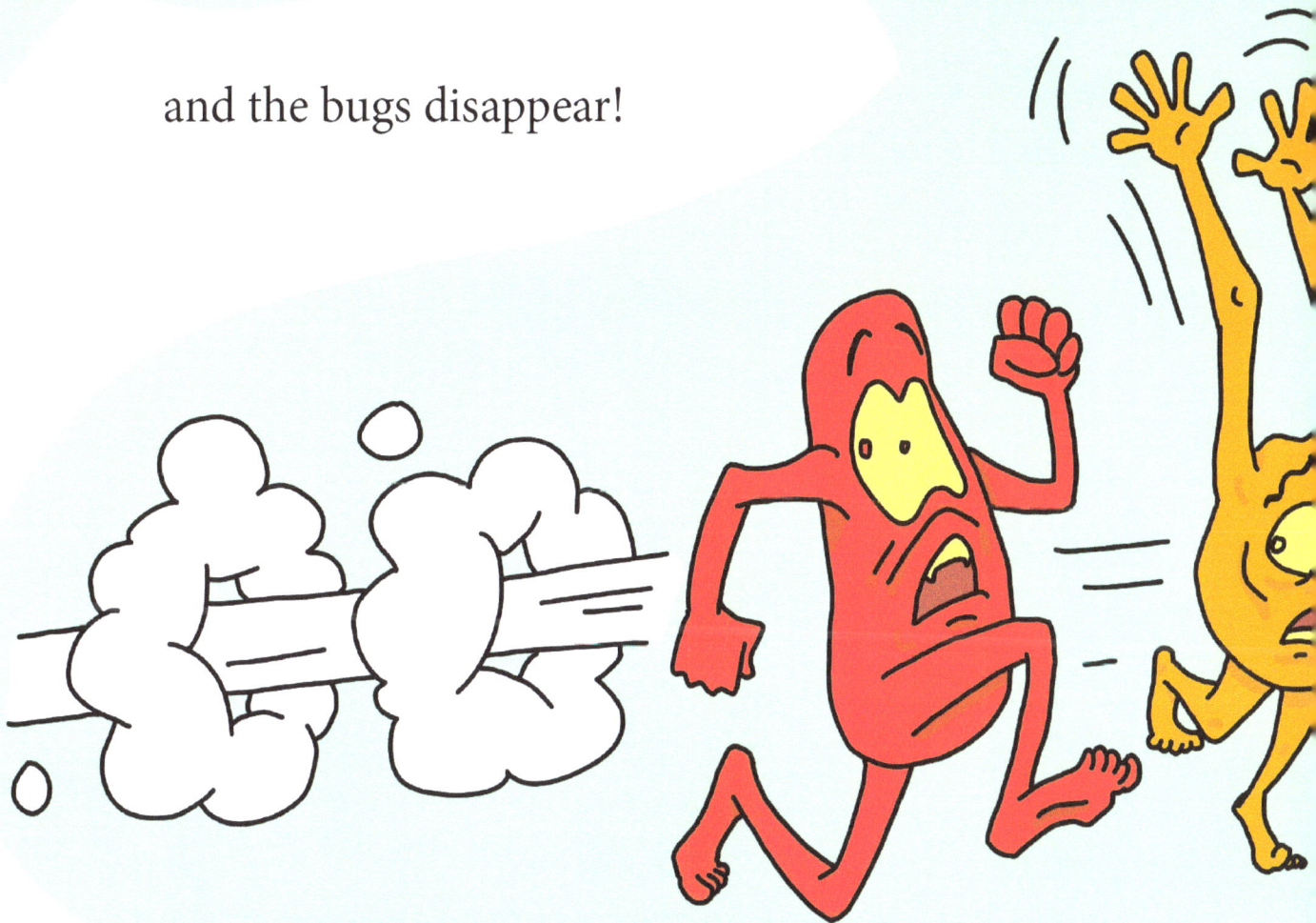

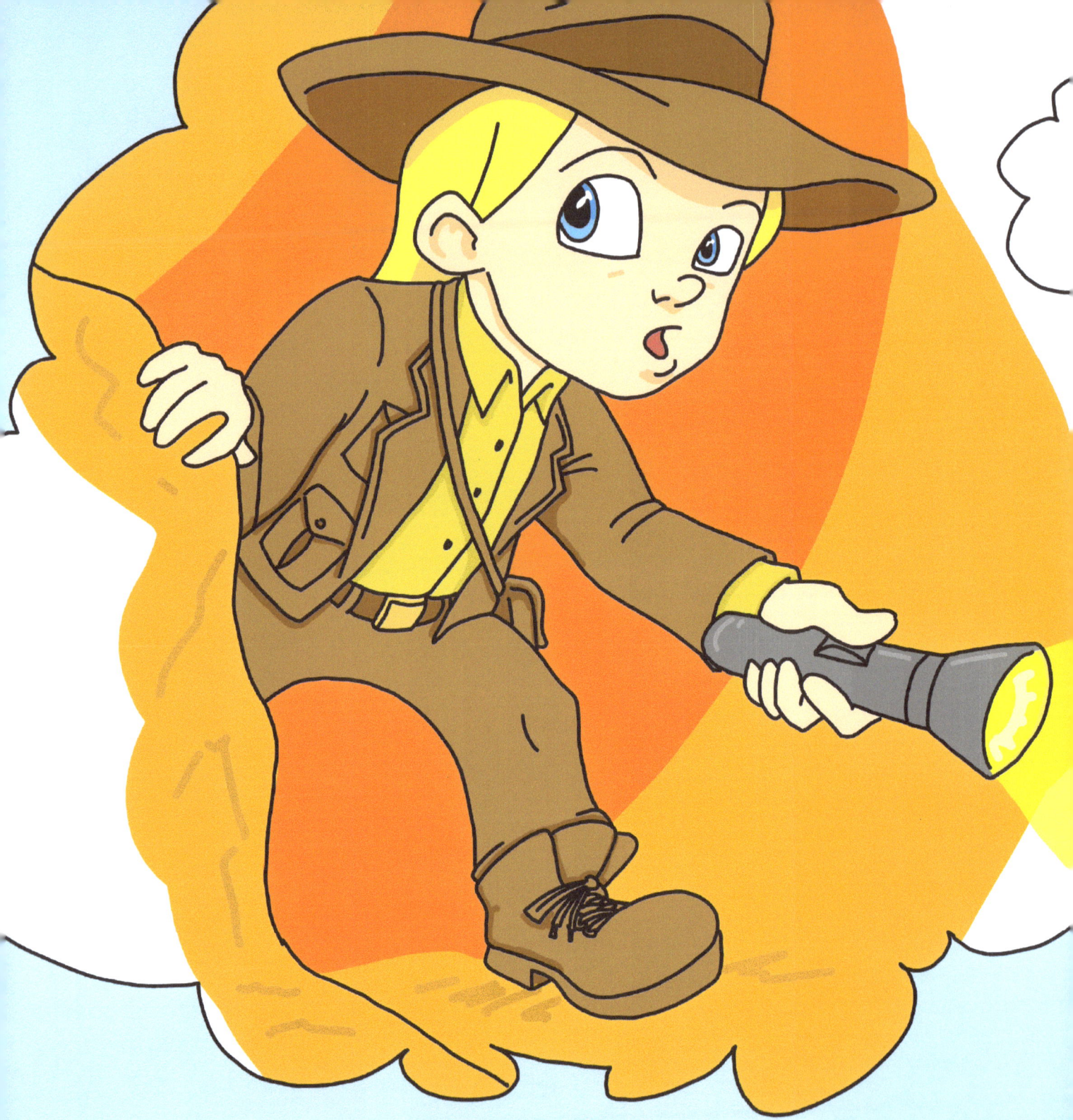

Juliette thought, "This science is cool!
"I'll never stop learning! I'm always in school!

"There are so many mysteries
still left to uncover.
"I wonder what's out there
for me to discover?"

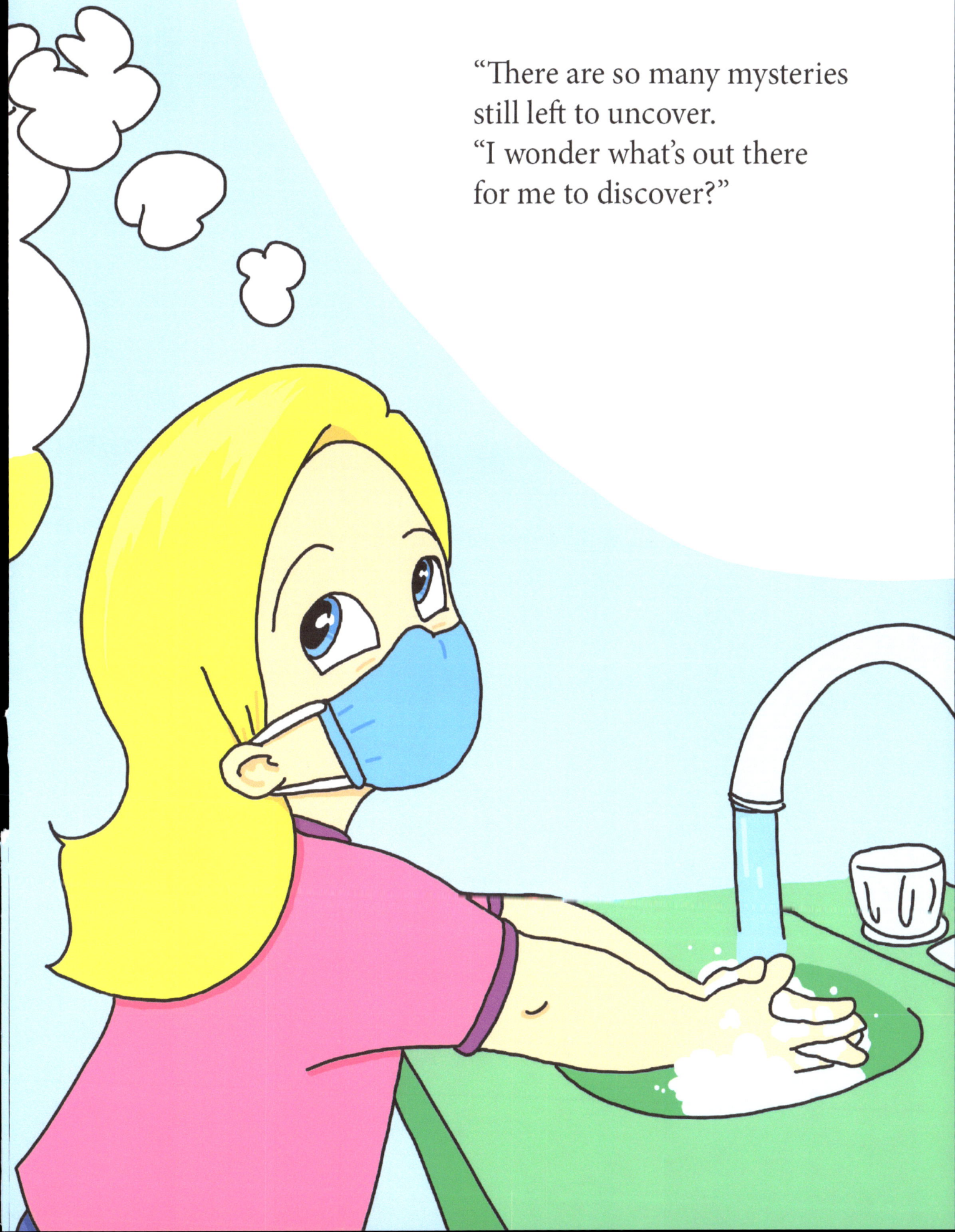

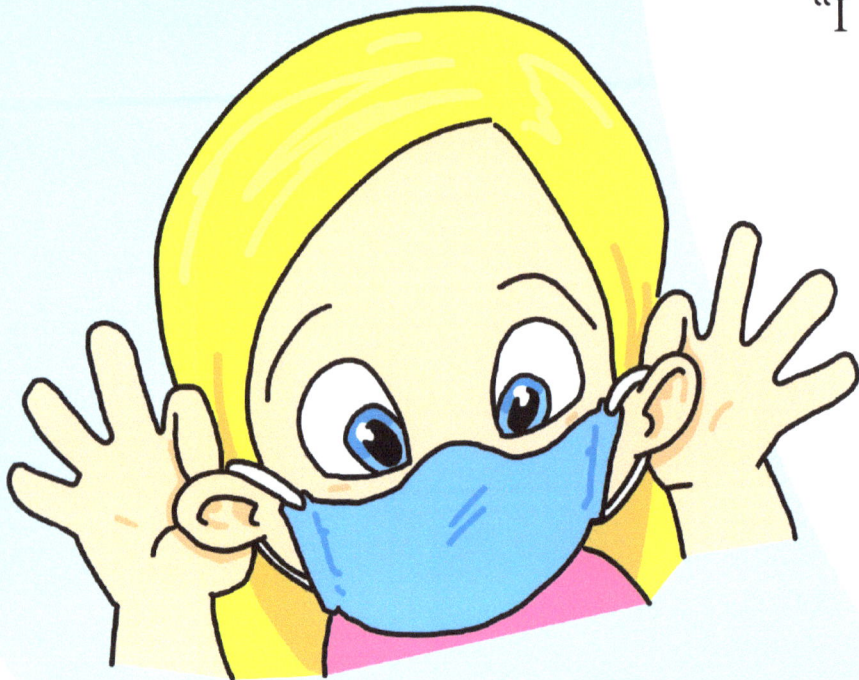

"I will still wear my mask,

wash my hands,

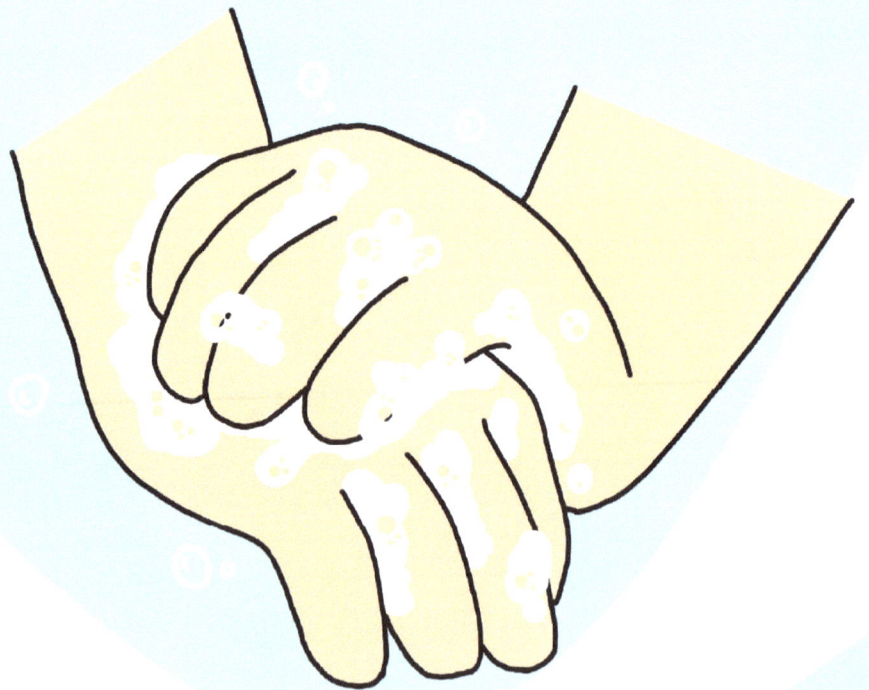

keep my distance.

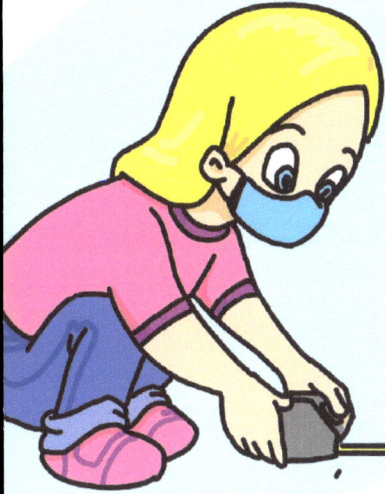

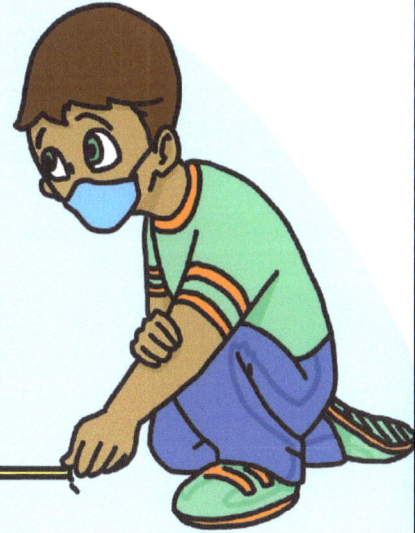

With the right vaccination,
I can build my resistance.

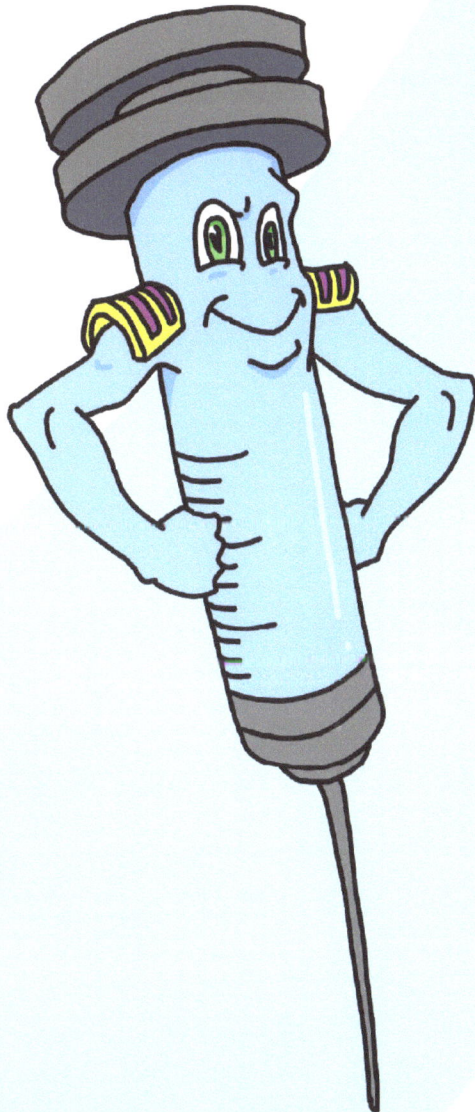

All of these things
are gifts I can share...

"To help those around me stay well and take care."

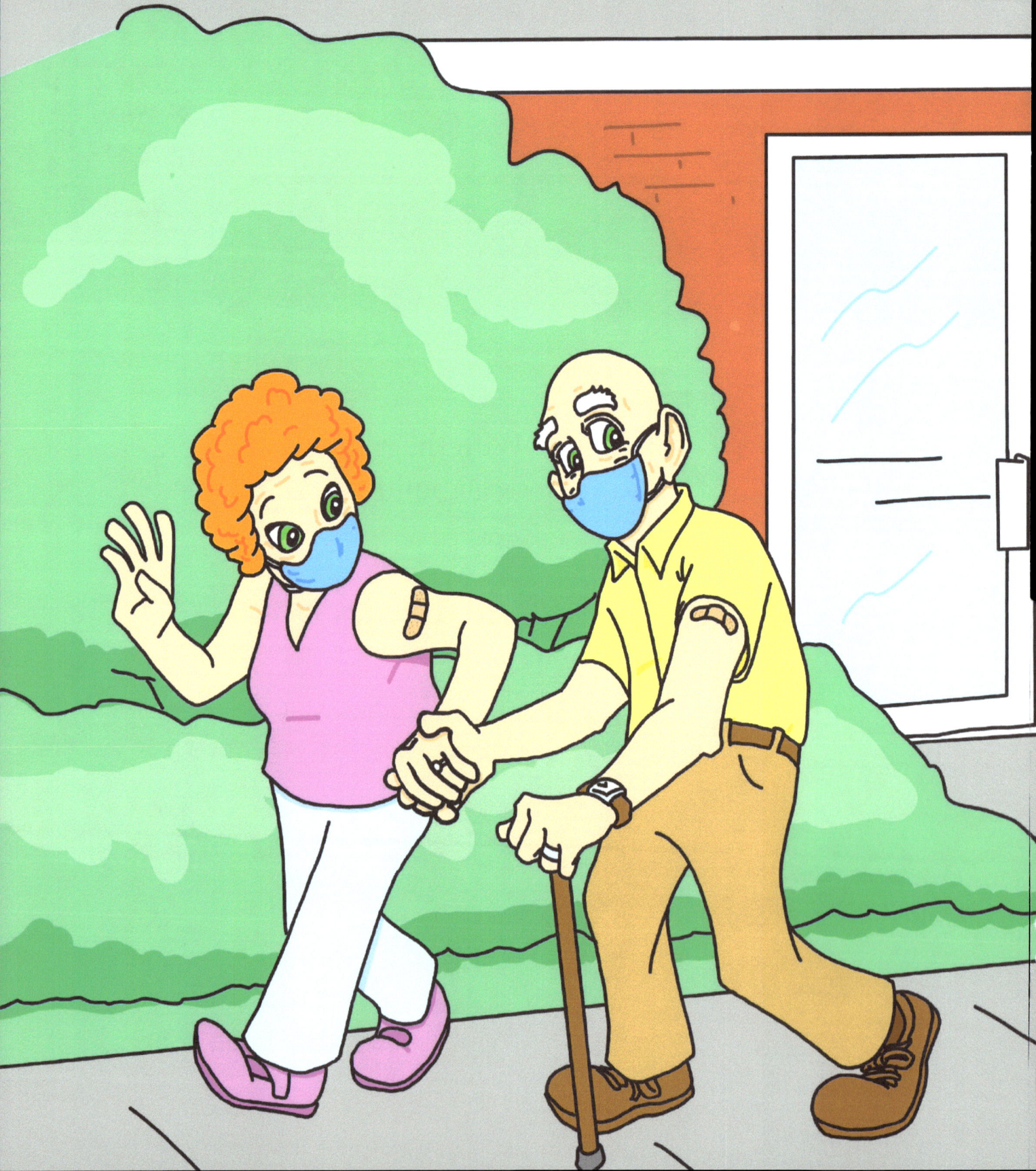

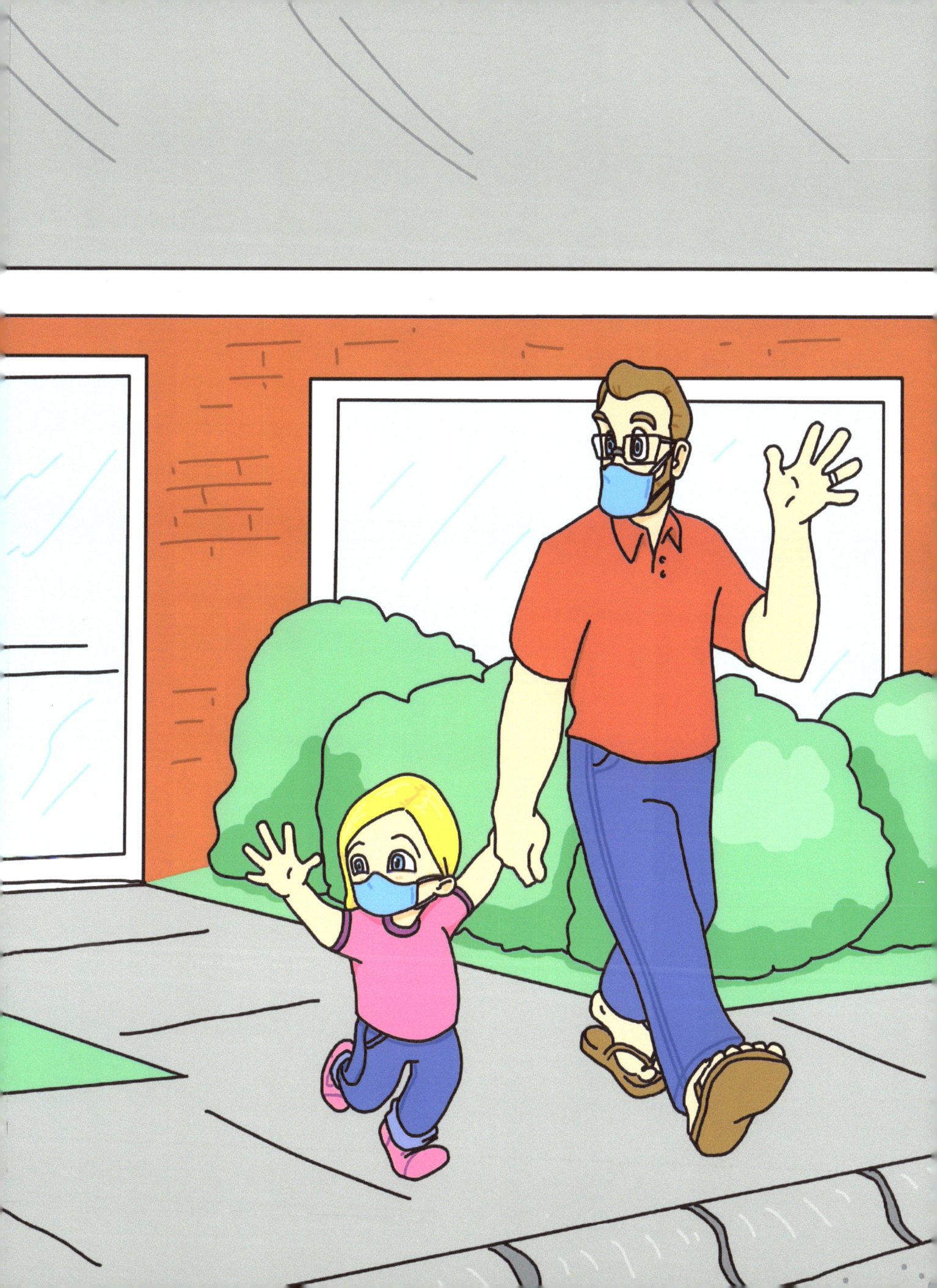

www.ingramcontent.com/pod-product-compliance
Lightning Source LLC
Chambersburg PA
CBHW060807270326
41927CB00003B/82